Let's TALK *About* DOWN THERE

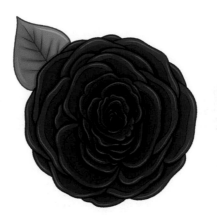

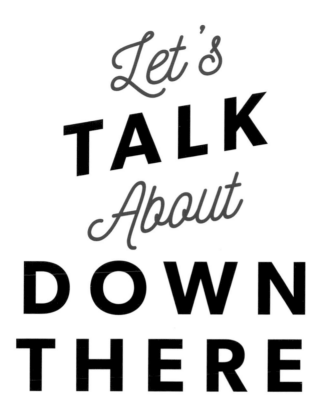

Let's TALK About DOWN THERE

An OB-GYN Answers All Your Burning Questions . . .
without Making You Feel Embarrassed for Asking

DR. JENNIFER LINCOLN, OB-GYN

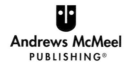

Andrews McMeel
PUBLISHING®

Andrews McMeel Publishing
a division of Andrews McMeel Universal
1130 Walnut Street, Kansas City, Missouri 64106

www.andrewsmcmeel.com

This book does not serve as a replacement for professional or medical advice or treatment. Readers should regularly consult medical professionals in matters relating to health and particularly with respect to any symptoms that may require diagnosis or medical attention. This book does not constitute a doctor–patient relationship. All opinions are the author's own.

21 22 23 24 25 TEN 10 9 8 7 6 5 4 3 2 1

ISBN: 978-1-5248-6576-4

Library of Congress Control Number: 2021934316

Illustrations by Charlotte Willcox

Editor: Allison Adler
Art Director: Holly Swayne
Production Editor: Elizabeth A. Garcia
Production Manager: Tamara Haus

Attention: Schools and Businesses
Andrews McMeel books are available at quantity discounts with bulk purchase for educational, business, or sales promotional use. For information, please e-mail the Andrews McMeel Publishing Special Sales Department: specialsales@amuniversal.com.

For my sons, who will grow up knowing that women can do anything.
For my husband, who believes the same.
For my parents, who told me this so I believed it too.

CONTENTS

CHAPTER 3
Facts for Feeling Good . . . 63

CHAPTER 6

Going to the Doctor . . . 135

CHAPTER 7

Possibly Pregnant . . . 157

INTRODUCTION

Hi! I'm Jen, aka Dr. Jennifer Lincoln. I'm a board-certified OB-GYN, and I like to talk about things that you might think are embarrassing, like vaginal and sexual health.

I talk about these things with my friends and my family. I post about them on Instagram. I set them to music on TikTok and hope that the audience there tolerates my videos (so far, they have).

For me, there's nothing embarrassing about answering questions about down there. I talk about vaginas and birth control like others talk about their new favorite coffee drink or the show they just spent all weekend binging—it's just a normal part of my day, and sometimes I could go on for hours.

Very few people get taught about how their bodies work, in school or elsewhere. I for sure fell into that category for most of my life. When your health class is taught by a nun, sometimes you don't ask all the questions you really want to. Am I right?

Before I did my medical training, I had a ton of unanswered questions, and I didn't really have a good place to get answers, which led to a lot of confusion and doubt.

I remember wishing that I had a place to ask those forbidden questions, a place where I could get medically accurate, evidence-based answers—free of judgment for asking them.

Every day at work I hope that my patients feel they have found that safe place in me. And on social media—where I spend so much of my time educating and myth-busting—I try to create the same environment.

I think I'm on to something, as evidenced by the over 1 million people who follow me on my social media channels and who send me messages daily saying that they finally feel like they understand their bodies. I have seen how hungry people are for facts and how desperate they are to fill in the gaps when it comes to how things down there work.

So, I decided to go one step further and write this book.

In these pages I hope you find the information you need. I also hope you'll find confidence, clarity, and the reassurance that you are normal and beautiful—just as you are.

I also hope you will feel included in this book, regardless of your gender identity. I have purposefully tried to use language inclusive to everyone. I recognize that the language may seem awkward at first, but my goal is to reach as many people as possible, especially those who have historically felt invisible within the discussion of these health care topics.

Another point I want to highlight is that I often use the word "doctor" or "OB-GYN" in this book. I do want to acknowledge that women's health care is a team sport. Family medicine physicians, nurse practitioners, physician assistants, midwives—they all are on the frontlines and providing this care, too, and I want to credit their roles as well.

This book is a place where shame, embarrassment, discrimination, and fear have no power.

I hope you enjoy.

CHAPTER 1

Period Puzzles

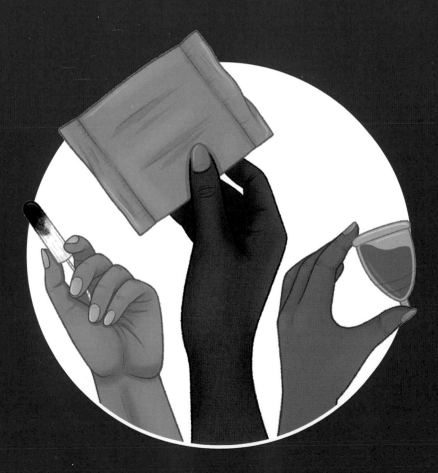

Does the color of my period `matter?`

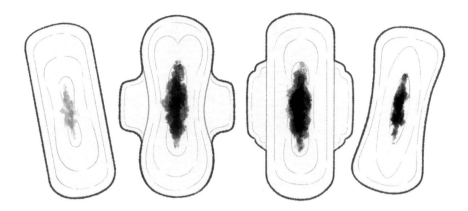

Period blood can be a few different hues, and that's totally normal.
The breakdown generally goes like this:

Pinkish: often spotting before the main period starts

Bright red: the main part of your period

Dark red, black: end of your period (older blood oxidizes in the uterus and is darker)

Brown: often seen at the very end of the period, more like a discharge or staining

That's really it.

Don't listen to "wellness experts" who may try to convince you that they can read your fortune by analyzing the color of your pad.

They claim dark blue or purple blood is from too much estrogen and you ARE IN DANGER, and light, wispy pink is from too little estrogen, which means you're deficient in vitamins and your adrenal glands aren't working.

But wait—there's more! These menstrual psychics also just happen to sell products that they claim will balance your hormones and make your periods a beautiful crimson red again. Are we surprised?! Buyer beware: Unfortunately, a lot of wellness and hormone "experts" try to suck you in by convincing you that you've got a problem and then selling you a pill or supplement that can "fix" it. Shady.

Let's put this myth in the trashcan where it belongs, next to your used pads and tampons.

Why is my period heavy and making me miserable?

Periods go by many names (Aunt Flo, the curse, crimson tide—so many euphemisms!), but if any of these describe yours, we need to talk: gushing, hemorrhage, tsunami of blood, cramps from hell, insides feel like they're being twisted in a vice, clots the size of a golf ball.

Ouch.

That's not normal.

> **MENORRHAGIA**
> the fancy word for a heavy period, also known as "heavy menstrual bleeding" in gynecologist language. What's heavy? If it seems heavy to you, that's good enough for us.
>
> **DYSMENORRHEA**
> painful periods.

If you're experiencing either of these and they are making it so you can't live your normal life during your period, it's time to chat with your friendly OB-GYN, because you don't have to live like this.

HERE'S A LIST OF THINGS THAT MIGHT BE AT PLAY:

Fibroids (benign balls of muscle and fibrous tissue that form in the uterus)

Polyps (small growths in the uterus or cervix that are often benign)

Adenomyosis (when the cells from the uterine lining that should bleed and shed each month instead grow deeper into the walls of the uterus)

Precancerous or cancerous growths (these are RARE in young women, so keep that in mind!)

Bleeding disorders (such as von Willebrand disease, when blood does not clot normally)

Hormonal issues (for example, thyroid dysfunction and polycystic ovarian syndrome aka PCOS)

Extremes of weight (too low or too high)

Stress

Infections (think gonorrhea, chlamydia, pelvic inflammatory disease)

Medications (blood thinners or even certain birth control like the copper IUD)

Endometriosis (when cells of the uterine lining are found outside the uterus and can cause inflammation and subsequent pain)

Cervical stenosis (if blood can't flow out of the uterus through the cervix, it can stretch your uterus—ouch!)

That's a lot, I know. Your doctor will target what they do based on what seems most likely. Based on your history and exam she may order bloodwork, an ultrasound or other imaging studies, send tests for infection or cancer, and maybe offer medications (like birth control) or surgery if she thinks it may help.

The good news is we have a LOT of treatments available to get you back to your regularly scheduled life.

What does it mean if I'm
bleeding in between my periods?

First, some definitions.

> **NORMAL MENSTRUAL CYCLE**
> lasts between 21 to 35 days, with bleeding lasting on
> average for 5 days. It is tracked as the first day of one period
> to the first day of the next period.
>
> **INTERMENSTRUAL BLEEDING**
> what we doctors call spotting or bleeding in between
> periods.

Intermenstrual bleeding can be caused by a few different things, and it is important to let your doctor know if it's happening to you so they can figure out why and then help make it go away—because who needs that annoyance in their life?

The good news is that usually bleeding in between periods is not life threatening and can be fixed. Hooray!

Let's break down what might be the culprit:

Hormonal	• Immature hormonal pathways when periods first start in teens (normal!) • PCOS (not ovulating regularly) • Thyroid issues • Nearing menopause (irregular ovulation as ovaries start to stop releasing eggs)
Anatomical	• Polyps • Fibroids • Precancerous/cancerous cells
Other	• Bleeding disorders • Medications (can be a normal side effect of some birth control) • Infections (especially sexually transmitted infections) • Trauma (sex can cause blood vessels in the vagina or on the cervix to break and bleed) • Skin disorders (e.g., fragile skin can tear)

I only have a few periods a year— is that OK?

The answer is . . . maybe, maybe not.

(Annoying answer, I know).

I want you to think of your period as a vital sign—if it doesn't happen regularly, that could be a sign your body is telling you something. As I've mentioned before, a period should last about five days, with the average cycle length between 21 to 35 days long. If your period doesn't fit those general outlines, we want to know.

OLIGOMENORRHEA
when a cycle is longer than 35 days.

HYPOTHALAMIC–PITUITARY–OVARIAN AXIS
the name for the structures in your body that all work together to release hormones that make you have a normal period. When you first begin menstruating, these structures are still figuring out the kinks—and that's why periods may be infrequent for a while.

Having skipped periods can put you at higher risk for having trouble conceiving down the road as well as precancerous changes and cancer of the uterus. That's why it's important to investigate whether there's an underlying issue or work to get them on track.

Skipping periods can be a sign of a few things. These include:

- Your period has just started and your body is adjusting (normal as a teen)
- Pregnancy (yes, this has to be ruled out!)
- PCOS
- Primary ovarian insufficiency (aka early menopause)

- Perimenopause (the years surrounding menopause before periods stop completely)
- Thyroid disorders
- Stress
- Excessive exercise
- Large fluctuations in weight
- High prolactin levels (from breastfeeding or tumors that make this hormone)
- Medications (birth control, certain psychiatric medications, and more)

Depending on the "why" of why your periods are few and far between, it may or may not be something to address. For example, if it's because of birth control, it is *totally* OK to skip your periods. That's actually a huge reason many women use it! But if it's from something like PCOS, skipping periods can actually be detrimental in the long term.

Is it true if I drink lots of water my period will be shorter?

If this were true, wouldn't we all just hook ourselves up to a hose every 28 days?

Sadly, this is a total myth, friends. But despite this claim having no data to support it, it has been shared oodles of times on social media.

I dove down the research rabbit hole (which was actually a rather short journey, since there was nothing to be found) to see where this idea came from. Mostly, I found mentions on "wellness" sites and in magazine articles that contained no references, so that's a red flag. One source claimed that if you don't drink enough water, your blood thickens. Therefore, drinking more water on your period will thin your blood, and it will "flush" out of your uterus faster.

Thankfully, this isn't true—our bodies are pretty savvy, and our blood doesn't turn to total sludge if we are thirsty.

Bottom line: Staying hydrated is always a good idea. On your period, being hydrated may help you experience fewer cramps (the uterus is a muscle, and dehydrated muscles can cramp more). But don't go overboard—just drink enough so that your urine is pale yellow. Stay away from the hose.

What do I do if my vagina smells during my period?

I want to make sure we acknowledge the vagina for what it is before we work on this one: a vagina.

It should smell like . . . a vagina.

And during your period, it's OK if that smell changes some.

Blood coming from the uterus and into the vagina is going to have a scent. It's going to alter the pH of the vagina a bit. That's totally normal.

If you notice a smell that you aren't a fan of, you may want to consider changing your menstrual products more frequently—this is especially true for pads. Or maybe you want to give up pads altogether and go with cups or tampons, since it's the blood sitting on the pad itself that can be causing the odor.

If you feel like things are really bad down there, PLEASE don't throw feminine washes, sprays, or douches at it. These products are terrible for your vagina, which doesn't need all those irritating fragrances and chemicals. In fact, using these products can actually throw off your pH and make you predisposed to infections—so you end up worse than before you started!

Worried about your scent? Come on in and see us in the office. We can figure out if there is an infection that needs to be treated (you can be more prone to infections on your period since your pH does normally vary slightly, which can help some bacteria thrive). Or maybe there's a tampon that was accidentally left in place for a few days (yes, this totally happens, and we will not judge you).

Before you worry: Yes, we can see you on your period. Our whole career involves various bodily fluids, and period blood doesn't scare us off.

Can I get pregnant on my period?

I can't tell you how many times I've been asked, "Can I get pregnant on day ___ of my cycle?"

The truth is that you are not fertile every waking moment of the month. Of course, we tend to err on the side of caution in sex ed class (if you even had one, that is) and even when I see you in the office when we are talking about pregnancy prevention.

In reality, you are fertile for about six days out of every normal, regularly timed menstrual cycle. This is called the "fertile window."

FERTILE WINDOW

usually the six days before you ovulate, ending on the day of ovulation. Within that, you are *most* fertile in the three days before ovulation.

The rest of the time within a normal cycle, pregnancy is highly unlikely.

But.

(There's always a "But.")

I can't 100 percent say you will never get pregnant on your period. That could be because what you might have called a period wasn't a period at all (maybe some spotting or bleeding from sex, for example), and so calculating when you ovulate in any given month is tricky. Or maybe you have short cycles, and having sex at the end of your period, combined with sperm being able to live for a few days, is close enough to when you ovulate in your next cycle.

To put it another way: If your risk of pregnancy on a certain day is only 1 percent, that still isn't a 100 percent guarantee of no pregnancy. Someone is going to get pregnant some of the time.

My recommendation: Don't rely on being on your period for birth control.

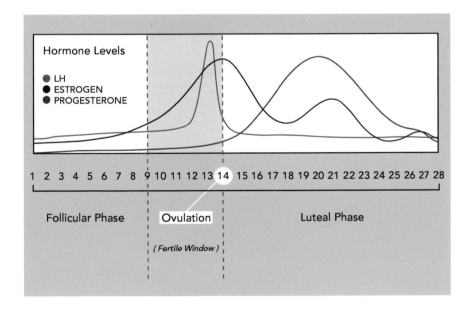

Can I have sex
on my period?

Absolutely!

If you want to have sex on your period, go for it. If you don't because it doesn't sound like fun or you don't feel up to it, that's OK too.

Only do it if you want to.

This is advice that applies to sex 24/7/365.

Some tips to help with period sex:

- Remove any tampons.
- Some menstrual cups are OK to leave in place and can contain the blood, so check to see if yours is one of them.
- Use sheets or a towel that you are OK getting blood on.
- Consider sex in the shower!
- Still use birth control (see above) and condoms to prevent STIs.
- If you usually use lube, you can likely skip it—menstrual blood helps to make things slippery.

I've heard periods are supposed to hurt. Is this true?

There are a lot of layers to this question. The idea that periods are *supposed* to hurt is one steeped in old misogynistic beliefs about people who menstruate being an inferior, dangerous sex whose sexuality needs to be controlled. How does society do that? We don't adequately teach people about their bodies, we make it hard for them to access care, and then we normalize pain as a way of keeping them in check.

Think about it. "Natural childbirth" without medical pain relief has been elevated to a godly place in mom circles. Periods that leave you incapacitated? Oh, honey, that's just your monthly curse. Take an ibuprofen and go back to class. No!

Hear me loud and clear: Yes, periods can be crampy because of an increase in prostaglandins (natural chemicals in your blood stream) that cause your uterus to contract and expel the menstrual blood. Sure, hormone fluctuations can leave you with some nausea, gas, looser poops, or constipation.

But should they cause you pain that disrupts your life? Should you have to take days off from work or school every month because you can't leave your bed? Hell to the no.

So if this is you, know you don't need to suffer, and we can work together to stop letting your period put the brakes on your life.

PERIODS THAT MAKE YOU CRY COULD BE SIGNS OF SOME OF THE FOLLOWING:
Endometriosis
Adenomyosis
Fibroids
Bleeding disorders
PCOS and hormone imbalances (e.g., thyroid disorders)
Ovarian cysts
Adhesions or scar tissue
Infections
Anatomical abnormalities
Precancerous or cancerous growths

Do I need
organic tampons?

Need? No.

OK to use? Sure.

If you are worried about organic versus conventional tampons, I first want us to take a step back and acknowledge that we are pretty privileged if this is a decision we get to consider. In the vast majority of developing countries, people who menstruate have very limited or no access to menstrual products. Because of this, they can't go to school or work during their period or they are shunned as being dirty a week out of every month.

Truly, the ability to purchase organic tampons is a privilege we need to acknowledge. Now let me get off my soapbox and answer your question.

Let's talk about claims and the realities of organic tampons. Keep in mind *both* are regulated as medical devices by the FDA:

CLAIM	REALITY CHECK
Organic tampons contain fewer dioxins (endocrine-disrupting and cancer-causing chemicals) than conventional tampons.	• Not true—negligible amounts are found in *both* kinds of tampons. • The amount of dioxins you are exposed to in tampons is 13,000–240,000 times *less* than what you are exposed to in food.
Conventional tampons have asbestos.	False.
Toxic shock syndrome (TSS) risk is higher when using conventional tampons.	False.
Organic tampons are better for the environment.	Arguable. Organic crops require more land and water to grow than conventional crops.

CLAIM	REALITY CHECK
Pesticide exposure is higher in conventional tampons.	• Maybe—but the FDA requires that tampons be free of pesticides to be approved. • Don't forget that organic farming still uses pesticides. • We need more data on exposure to *both* classes of tampons.
Organic tampons are more expensive.	This is a fact for some brands.

At the end of the day, pick whichever one makes you happy. Avoid scents and fragrances in all cases. And if you find your vagina is happier with an organic tampon, that is perfectly OK. But if your wallet isn't, don't feel guilty about switching.

My parents won't let me get on any birth control for my period.
What now?

It can be really challenging when you want to care for your body but encounter obstacles along the way.

First, I would suggest that you ask your parents to level with you—why don't they want you on birth control? Is it because they are worried about side effects? Do they think it means you will start having sex because of it? Something else?

Then (if you feel like you can do this) I think it is great when a person who wants to use BC makes an appointment with the OB-GYN *with* their reluctant parent so that we can all have one informative conversation together. Your OB-GYN can discuss risks and benefits and address any concerns. Your parents may not even realize that many women are prescribed birth control to treat many medical issues, and it isn't *all* about pregnancy prevention. You'd be surprised how good and productive these visits can be!

Still struggling with getting your parents on board and want to access BC confidentially? Check out page 106, where I discuss different options.

Are menstrual cups
OK?

Yes, with a small caveat: If you have an IUD in place, there is some data that shows using a menstrual cup may increase your risk for the IUD expelling, or accidentally coming out. This doesn't mean you absolutely *can't* use both an IUD and a menstrual cup, but it's something to discuss with your doctor. Of note, the cups used in these studies relied on suction to remain in place, so one cup option that may be better for IUD users is one that does not use any suction. The good news is that with the progesterone IUDs, periods can be so light or absent that a cup isn't even needed—hooray! We can't say the same about the copper IUD though, which can lead to heavier periods for some women.

If you're worried about increased risk of infections like toxic shock syndrome or yeast infections with menstrual cups, you can rest easy. Studies have shown infection rates are the same (and maybe lower!) when compared to pads and tampons.

There are literally hundreds of cups out there, and it can be hard to know where to start. Sometimes it's about trial and error and an adjustment period while you learn to use them, but if you're excited about saving money and helping the environment, a cup might be the right choice for you.

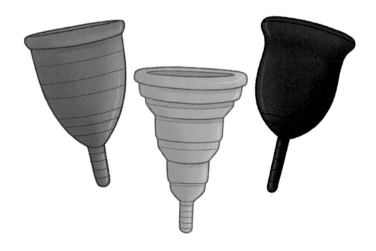

Are cloth pads
OK to use?

Cloth pads are the adult version of cloth diapers: reusable absorbent products that you can wash and reuse. You can feel happy about saving the earth and saving money (in the long run, that is, as they are more of an investment up front) if this is your preferred period protection.

But is it safe to have blood-soaked cloth in your underwear for hours at a time? Won't bacteria breed and make you prone to infections? Is this some new trend that is just a fad?

First, to the fad question: Cloth pads may seem unfamiliar to those of us in developed countries, but these products have been used for a long time in places where access to menstrual products is scarce, and they used to be commonplace here too. Not all people can afford pads or tampons every month, and some instead use some kind of cloth pad. Heck, it's where the term "being on the rag" came from!

These products are generally fine to use. As long as you change them when you need to, you should be OK. It is true that the cloth might not wick away as much moisture from your skin like a disposable pad does, but you can manage that with more frequent changes.

Of course, if you do notice any skin sensitivities or new infections, then they might not be the best product for you.

Are period underwear **gross?**

> **MENSTRUAL UNDERWEAR**
> reusable underwear that has an absorbent area where period blood collects.

I don't think they are, and I am *really* jealous these products weren't around when I first started my period.

Remember how you lived in fear that you'd get your period at school, where periods were barely discussed and you knew a period stain would be like the scarlet letter on the back of your uniform? No? That was just me? Anyway . . .

. . . how nice would it have been to have had period underwear to wear just in case? So jealous.

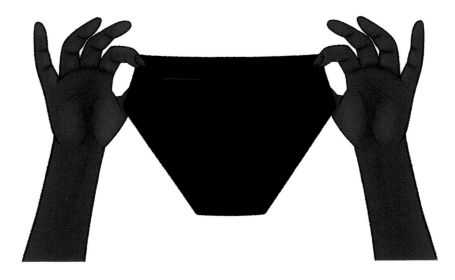

But back to the question: No, it's not gross, and it's another option for menstruating folks or those about to menstruate, and I *love* having more options. They can be used alone or as a back-up for overflowing pads or tampons.

There are many types on the market, and they all vary in how they are made and how much they absorb. Some have antimicrobial layers (some have silver fibers sewn in for this purpose). They can be expensive at the outset but can save money through repeated use.

Just like with anything else on your vulva, watch out for irritation. If you have concerns, consider trying something else when on your period to rule out menstrual underwear as the cause. And as always, if you aren't sure, ask your doctor.

Why is my period
late?

It can be super anxiety-provoking when your period fails to show up at its scheduled time. Where has it gone? When will it come back? And of course: AM I PREGNANT?!

It takes thousands of hormonal pathways and signals to make a period happen. Any disruption along the way can throw a monkey wrench in the process. So, yes, by all means make sure you aren't pregnant—but don't neglect to look at the other things that could be to blame:

- Stress
- Sleep disturbances
- Weight loss/gain
- Excessive exercise
- Breastfeeding
- Pituitary tumors
- Dietary changes
- Medications
- Birth control (totally OK to not have a period when on BC, FYI!)
- PCOS
- Thyroid disorders
- Diabetes
- Other autoimmune disorders like celiac disease
- Early menopause

If your period is nowhere to be seen for more than two to three months, let your doctor know. They will likely ask you to track your cycle (or lack thereof) as well as any other symptoms you've noticed and have you come in to figure out what kind of workup may be needed.

Is PMDD
a real thing?

Yes! And if you haven't heard about it till now, that's OK. Not everyone has, and I think it's important to talk about because many people are suffering unnecessarily.

Think of PMDD as PMS on steroids.

	PMS	PMDD
AKA	Premenstrual syndrome	Premenstrual dysphoric disorder
Stats	Affects 30–80% of people who menstruate	Affects 3–8% of people who menstruate
Symptoms	Psychological symptoms <ul><li>Anger/irritability</li><li>Anxiety</li><li>Depression</li><li>Feeling overwhelmed</li></ul> Physical symptoms <ul><li>Bloating</li><li>Increased appetite</li><li>Breast tenderness</li><li>Headaches</li><li>Fatigue</li><li>Muscle aches</li><li>Poor concentration</li></ul>	<ul><li>A more severe form of PMS symptoms, with significant mood disturbance (e.g., acute irritability that is somewhat disabling)</li><li>Interferes with your social life and your work</li></ul>
When	They both usually show up 1–2 weeks before your period and get better in the first few days of your period.	
Why	We think it's due to sensitivity to the fluctuations in the hormones that happen before you have a period.	

Worried you have PMS or PMDD? Track your symptoms (there are lots of great apps that make this easy to do). Bring the hard data to your doctor who can review it. It's important to know other things that need to be ruled out too, like depression, anxiety, and thyroid issues, so don't be surprised if your doctor wants to do some testing.

Good news: treatments exist! A combo of some of the following may be recommended if you are diagnosed with PMDD:

- Regular aerobic exercise
- Diet changes
- Eliminating caffeine, alcohol, etc., may help—but if no improvement is noted, feel free to add back!
- 1,200 mg calcium per day has been shown to help
- Herbal remedies (inconclusive evidence)
- Light therapy
- Behavioral therapy
- SSRI antidepressants
- Suppressing ovulation (birth control pills are the most studied, but other forms likely help too)

How do I
track my period?

Nowadays with so many apps made just for this purpose, tracking your period has never been easier. I'd say it's a big step up from using a paper planner and counting out the days like I had to (I'm aging myself . . .)!

Most apps will remind you to track and make it easy to log things like spotting and bleeding as well as period symptoms like cramping, bloating, and mood symptoms to give you an idea of how your cycle is affecting you.

Some tracking tips:

- Your first day of bright-red, full-flow bleeding is considered the first day of your period.
- Your cycle length is from the first day of one period to the first day of the next.
- No need to pay for a tracking app—lots of great free versions exist.

This data can actually be really useful if you have concerns about irregular or painful periods or concerns about PMS—you can show your doctor who can quickly see what your cycles look like for you and compare that info with the symptoms you are having.

CHAPTER 2

Care and Curiosities for Down There

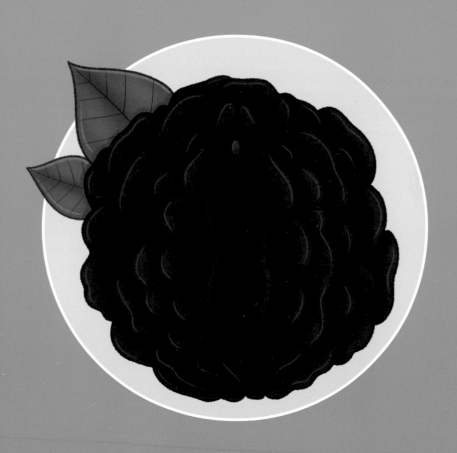

Why am I
always wet?

You can thank your vaginal discharge for the wetness you are feeling. It might feel gross to have wet underwear or discharge that is a bit slimy, but it totally has a purpose.

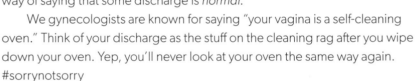

We even have an official name for this: physiological discharge.

Merriam-Webster defines "physiological" as "characteristic of or appropriate to an organism's healthy or normal functioning." This is a really wordy way of saying that some discharge is *normal*.

We gynecologists are known for saying "your vagina is a self-cleaning oven." Think of your discharge as the stuff on the cleaning rag after you wipe down your oven. Yep, you'll never look at your oven the same way again. #sorrynotsorry

Vaginal discharge is made up of mucous, fluid, and cells that have sloughed off from the cervix and vagina. It often has a watery or creamy consistency. How it appears and how much you have changes over the course of your menstrual cycle because of fluctuating hormone levels. Some people with vaginas have it daily, while others just notice it at certain times in their cycle. Up to a teaspoon over the course of a day is totally normal.

If you looked at your discharge under a microscope (I wouldn't judge you; I think it's cool), you'd see epithelial—aka mucosal lining—cells along with little bacteria that are a mix of types but often mostly the lactobacillus species. These are the good bacteria that keep your vaginal pH happy.

Not all discharge is good, though, and I'll explain what to look out for on page 32.

Last point: If you are worried about how much discharge you are having, or if you think it might be urine leaking, don't hesitate to talk with your doctor.

What does normal vaginal discharge look like?

Normal—physiological, remember?—vaginal discharge is often white, off-white, or clear in color. As I mentioned above, the appearance can vary throughout your menstrual cycle. It can be thin, creamy, gooey, and elastic, and it is usually a combination of all of these throughout your cycle.

Puberty is when most people will start to notice this discharge, and that's because the increased estrogen in their bodies during this time changes their vaginal mucosa and ecosystem. Then during menopause, there is less discharge for the opposite reason: lower estrogen levels.

Some people even use the appearance of their vaginal discharge to track their fertility. Cervical mucus changes throughout a menstrual cycle, and by checking the discharge at their vaginal opening, they can guess when they are most or least fertile. See the drawing below for a better idea of what this means:

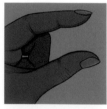

Dry: usually right after your period

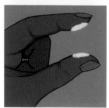

Thick or sticky (like glue): before and after ovulation, low fertility

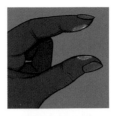

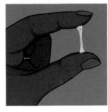

Clear and wet (like water): pre-ovulation, more fertile

Clear, stretchy (like egg white): ovulation, most fertile

Be warned that relying *only* on your vaginal discharge to predict when you will or won't get pregnant is not recommended for most people. It can take a few months to become familiar with your body, and up to 24 percent of people assigned female at birth can actually become pregnant using this as part of the Fertility Awareness Method within the first year of using it.

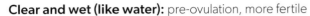

FERTILITY AWARENESS METHOD

a way to use various markers (such as body temperature, cervical mucus, and calendar charting) to try to predict when a person is most or least likely to get pregnant. This can be used when trying to conceive and also as a method of birth control.

How do I know if there's a problem
with my discharge?

Not all discharge is created equal.

If you notice any of the following, you should reach out to your doctor to get it checked out:

Color	green, dark yellow, gray, resembling pus
Odor	strong or foul odor
Consistency	foamy, lumpy like cottage cheese, or very thin with different coloring
Other symptoms	vulvar itching or burning, vulvar redness or swelling

Here are some examples of what could be going on:
- Bacterial vaginosis
- Yeast infection
- Trichomoniasis
- Gonorrhea
- Chlamydia
- Desquamative inflammatory vaginitis
- Something left in the vagina (e.g., tampon)

If you're experiencing this kind of discharge, I highly encourage you *not* to run to your nearest drugstore and self-treat. I know it's tempting. Who has time to go to the doctor? Why spend the money on a co-pay? I've been there, and I promise I hear you.

And yet . . . this is why I ask you to come in anyway:
- It can be hard to self-diagnose and know what you are treating.
- Lots of products in the feminine hygiene aisle are *not* recommended by doctors (despite what they may say on the label).

- These products often do more harm than good.
- Then when we do see you, you may have a more complicated issue than you had originally.

When you come in, we'll get a thorough history and do an exam that may include testing for infection, checking your vaginal pH, and looking at the discharge under the microscope. You'll leave with your questions answered, a medically sound treatment plan, and you and your discharge will be on the path to getting back on track!

I have too much discharge.
How do I decrease it?

OK, first I am going to ask that you read the topics earlier in this chapter. Quick recap: Vaginal discharge has a purpose!

Still worried? See your doctor. Make sure there isn't something treatable going on.

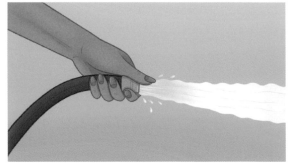

Still worried after that? Let me ask you this: Is someone making you feel bad about your discharge? Is your partner saying you are too wet or it's too much and they think it's gross? If that's the case, please tell them reading this book is their homework and it's due ASAP. You are also free to tell them "bye" from me because no one should shame you for your normal bodily functions.

If it's none of the above and you are still stressed, you can try the following:

- Change up your underwear: Undyed cotton tends to be more breathable and more absorbent than synthetic fibers.
- Change your underwear throughout the day.
- Consider skipping the pantyliners: If you like them, no need to stop (though no fragrances, please!), but sometimes the liners *cause* issues because your discharge sits there against your skin, leading to more vaginal moisture and maybe even *more* discharge.
- Use a menstrual cup: Yes, you can use it when not on your period! Just be sure to change it frequently and don't forget it is in there.
- Assess your vaginal routine: Are you using feminine washes, sprays, douches, or soaps with lots of fragrances in your sensitive vagina? Sometimes those are the culprit. Don't worry; we cover what is good to use on page 37.

How do I make my . . . ahem . . .
taste better?

Call me simple or old, but I didn't realize this was a thing until I joined TikTok. Who knew so many "protocols" existed for vaginal flavoring, from eating pineapple to drinking lemon juice? Not this gynecologist!

First: Outside of treating an infection, you don't need to do anything to change your vaginal odor or scent. If someone has complaints in that department, maybe it's time to call security and escort them out.

Second: This is 100 percent not a thing.

Google this and you'll see lots of articles that claim this is true (and this is why friends don't let friends indiscriminately google). But tell me, how the heck is a piece of pineapple going to survive the journey through your mouth, stomach, and intestines—with all the digestion that happens—and somehow secrete enough intact pineapple flavor by the time it "gets to" the vagina to cause any kind of change? And how come there is no data to show this is true?

It doesn't, and there is none.

Some things *do* cause changes in bodily scents or tastes—a classic example of this is changes to breast milk flavoring based on what mom eats (fun fact: this actually has an evolutionary purpose in that it exposes a baby to tastes they will eat as they grow up), but pineapple isn't going to change the way your vagina tastes or smells.

If you want to do this because you think it works for you, sure, go for it. If nothing else, pineapple is a good source of vitamin C. It isn't harmful unless you are purposely avoiding foods you love or forcing yourself to eat something you don't like because of an urban legend.

But I ask that you step back and think about why you feel you need to do anything to your vagina in the first place. Vaginas should smell and taste like vaginas. End of story.

What soap is best
to clean my vagina?

The following are the Ten Commandments of Cleaning Down There. Please memorize and follow accordingly.

1. Thou shalt not clean *inside* the vagina, as it is a self-cleaning entity and requires no assistance with its holy work.
2. Thou shalt remember that a vagina should smell like a vagina and not "summer romance."
3. Thou shalt not use feminine washes as they can kill off the good bacteria of your vagina, irritate your vulva, and give money to companies that make women feel dirty.
4. Thou shalt avoid feminine wipes for the same reasons as Commandment #3.
5. Thou shalt never douche, as douching can cause skin irritation, allergic reactions, and make you more susceptible to vaginal infections and STIs.

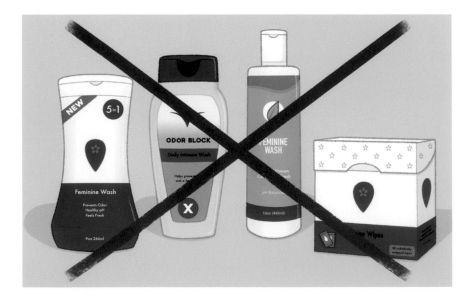

6. Thou shalt only ever cleanse the outside of the labia.
7. Thou shalt start with water, as many women only need this.
8. If more cleansing is desired, though shalt use cleansers without fragrances, dyes, or essential oils.
9. Thou shalt use cleansers that are close to a vagina's pH so the good bacteria there remain happy and healthy.
10. Thou shalt try scent-free soaps with caution, as soaps can be drying.

INGREDIENTS TO AVOID	GOOD BRANDS
Fragrance and perfumes	Vanicream Free & Clear
Essential oils	Cetaphil Gentle
Dyes	CeraVe
Parabens	Eucerin
Phthalates	Dove sensitive skin
Benzocaine	Dr. Bronner's unscented baby soap

Can I
douche?

You can, but I (and all evidence-based doctors) don't recommend it.

Society tells us the vagina is smelly and dirty and needs to be cleaned. This is false.

The vagina is a self-cleaning oven. I feel like a broken record in saying that, but it's important. The vaginal discharge that you have is the way in which your vagina flushes out dead cells and bacteria—completely without any assistance.

Douches (solutions varying from vinegar to chemical-laden feminine washes to bleach—YES, *BLEACH*) are completely unnecessary.

Douches can:

- Kill off the good microorganisms in your vagina
- Throw off your vaginal pH
- Cause irritation, allergic reactions, and burns to your sensitive skin down there
- Make you more prone to vaginal infections
- Cause vaginal dryness

Despite this, one in five American women still douche. It's hard to break vaginal shame culture.

When you buy a douche product, you are not only spending your money that could have gone to something more fun (Coffee! A pedicure! Literally anything!), you are also giving money to the feminine hygiene industry, which profits off of making us feel dirty and shameful. I don't think they deserve one more penny.

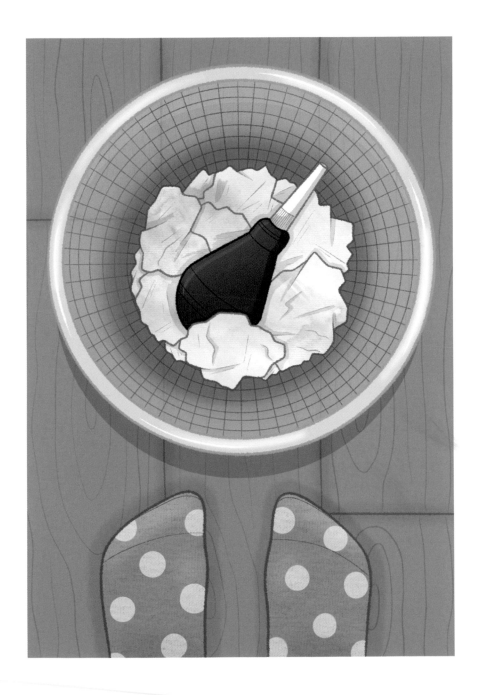

How do I fix the
pH of my vagina?

I get this question a lot, and I always ask back, "Why do you think something is wrong with it?"

Some people with vaginas are worried about discharge or odor—and that is a totally valid concern—but others think they have to "do" something to keep their pH healthy even when nothing seems off.

The good news is that your vagina is usually pretty good about regulating itself. The normal vaginal pH is 3.8–4.5, which is an acidic environment. That is because the bacteria in the vagina called lactobacilli (the dominant bacteria found there after puberty starts) produce lactic acid. That acid is what sets the pH.

If there are no problems or concerns about infection, there is nothing you need to do to regulate your vaginal pH. Your vagina has this one covered.

I know it's confusing because we see *so many* products that are advertised to address this—soaps and washes that promise to "balance" your pH, or probiotics, supplements, suppositories, or yogurts that claim they will help maintain a "healthy vaginal environment."

If you are worried about your vagina and its pH, see your doctor first, since they can actually test your pH and determine if anything is in fact out of balance. But outside of that, there's no need to manage your vaginal pH. And using these products can do the exact opposite of what they claim and cause more problems than they fix.

We have enough things to worry about in life—no need to add imaginary problems to the list!

Can steaming help
my vagina?

Not everyone has heard of vaginal steaming, so let me explain this one first.

> **VAGINAL STEAMING**
> also called v-steaming or yoni steaming, is the process of adding herbs to water that is then heated to a steaming temperature. A person then sits over this water with the goal that the steam goes up into their vagina and uterus.

This has been practiced in some Asian and African cultures for centuries and became more visible after Gwyneth Paltrow endorsed it on her website in 2015. Oh, Gwyneth.

Why v-steam? Supporters claim that benefits include postpartum healing, tightening the vagina, keeping the vagina "fresh," vaginal "detoxification," promoting fertility, healing fibroids, lessening menstrual cramps, increasing your sex drive, reducing stress, revitalizing your uterus . . . I mean, really, who doesn't want all that?!

It sounds great, but, unfortunately, there is no data to support any of this. It also doesn't make biological sense. How does hot water with mugwort and rosemary make your vagina tighter?

I have been told that, as a physician, I should not come out against something that has been so important to other cultures and especially not something with the goal of celebrating womanhood. I've been told there is no harm, so why belittle a practice that many enjoy?

Unfortunately, it's not harmless. People have suffered burns requiring reconstructive surgery from this practice. That's pretty bad.

While that sucks, what bothers me most is that practices like this are rooted in the idea that vaginas are dirty or broken and need to be fixed or freshened.

In my mind, this belongs in the same category as the whole feminine hygiene industry—one that profits off of making people feel bad about themselves.

Not to mention that these practices can actually throw off a vagina's pH and lead to overgrowth of harmful bacteria and can also delay care for legitimate medical problems like painful sex, miserable periods, or infertility.

There have been *lots* of cultural practices through the ages that we eventually discarded as we realized that they didn't work or that they caused harm. I'd love to see this one go that way and instead be replaced by something that honors just how amazing vaginas are without the aid of "cleansers," even herbal ones.

Yoni eggs and yoni pearls:
yay or nay?

I thought we were going to stop at vaginal steaming, but it seems we've got more to talk about when it comes to putting things in your vagina. Call me sheltered, but yoni eggs and yoni pearls were not covered in any of my medical training, and maybe you haven't heard of them either. Let's review.

YONI EGGS
polished eggs made out of jade and other stones that are supposed to be placed in the vagina. There have been claims that these restore your energy, heal your chakras, make you more fertile, transform you spiritually and sexually, strengthen your pelvic floor, and more. We again have Gwyneth to thank for making this one popular.

YONI PEARLS
small, cloth-covered balls containing herbs wrapped in mesh that are inserted into the vagina and left there for up to a day or longer with the goal of cleaning or "detoxing" your vagina from toxins. They are supposed to treat fibroids, cramps, infertility, PCOS, endometriosis, infections, tighten your vagina, and more. WOW!

I wish all those claims were true, but, once again, they lack any scientific evidence supporting them. Even claims that yoni eggs are part of an ancient Chinese practice have been debunked. The multiple videos on social media showing all the "toxins" that came out when yoni pearls were removed are just showing the terrible inflammation and increased discharge that result from this product's use.

And, yes, harm exists. Porous eggs left in the vagina can absorb bacteria and give you an infection rather than curing one. Herbal packets that are left in the vagina for days at a time may increase your risk of toxic shock syndrome, bacterial vaginosis, and contact dermatitis.

Ask yourself: Who is making these claims? Are they trying to sell you something? Are they convincing you that you are dirty without their product? Don't believe them. Be ever vigilant.

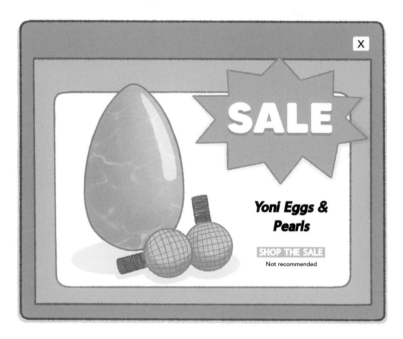

What is the best way to
remove my pubic hair?

It is OK to want to remove your pubic hair, but it is 100 percent a personal grooming decision. There is no medical reason to do this.

And it's really important to understand that pubic hair has a purpose. Did you know that your pubic hair . . .

- Protects your sensitive vulvar skin by reducing chafing and microabrasions?
- Helps to maintain the good-for-you bacteria?
- Blocks bacteria and other icky things from going into your vagina?

It really is there for a reason.

Our culture has decided that, for the most part, pubic hair should be removed. The pornography industry has normalized adults being completely bare down there when this is absolutely not the biological norm at all.

If you decide you do want to remove your pubic hair, know that it puts you at increased risk for sexually transmitted infections and skin infections *no matter how you do it*. Think long and hard whether or not you want to do it, and if the answer is still yes, check out the good and the bad of each of these methods on the following pages:

	HOW IT WORKS	POSITIVES	NEGATIVES	MY TIPS
Trimming	Scissors or electric clippers shorten the hair	Lower chance of skin injury or infection	Doesn't remove hair entirely	This is a great, low-risk way to remove pubic hair, especially if you just want to trim the bikini line.
Shaving	Razor blades physically remove hair	• More affordable • Doesn't require any salon or office visits	Risk of ingrown hairs, infection, skin lacerations, and injury	• Shower first. • Use a new razor blade each time—ideally a single blade. • Use a fragrance-free cream or gel to help the razor glide. • Shave in the direction the hair grows. • Don't pull the skin taut while shaving. • Apply a fragrance-free moisturizer afterward.
Waxing or sugaring	Sticky substance is applied to the hair follicle, which is then pulled off	• Lasts longer than shaving • Hair regrowth is less itchy	• Same risks as shaving • Possible skin burns • Potential for irritation/allergic reaction	• Go to a salon that has good hygiene practices. • Make sure they use new wooden applicators for each application—no double-dipping! • Test the temperature of the wax on a warm patch of skin first.

	HOW IT WORKS	POSITIVES	NEGATIVES	MY TIPS
Chemical depilatories aka Nair, Veet, Magic Shaving Powder	Chemicals dissolve the hair, which is then wiped off	I can't think of any.	These products are known for concerning chemical burns and skin irritation and allergic reactions.	Avoid!
Laser	Delivers mild radiation to hair follicles	Permanent or semi-permanent over multiple sessions.	• Costly • Requires multiple sessions • Not able to be done on all hair types or colors • Can cause skin redness, swelling, discoloration, blistering, scarring	You're safest in the hands of a trained professional, like a plastic surgeon or dermatologist.
Electrolysis	Involves inserting a probe into the hair follicle and sending an electric current through it	• Truly permanent • Works on any hair type or color	• Costly • Requires multiple sessions • Risk of scarring or infection • Can be painful	Go to a board-certified dermatologist.

My partner says my vagina smells funny—
what could it be?

Let's get this out of the way: Your partner should be thanking their lucky stars they even get to be NEAR your vagina. So. Let's first acknowledge that and decide whether or not they get to see it again.

But to answer your question: Vaginas are supposed to smell like . . . vaginas.

Not roses, or "morning paradise," or whatever other fragrance feminine-wash companies are trying to sell you (also: what does morning paradise *actually* smell like??).

Go back to page 32 to read more about discharge. Decide if your discharge might have an odor that could be from an infection. If so—see your doc. If not, feel reassured that your vagina is happy—and your partner should be too.

Should I take probiotics
to keep my vagina healthy?

With the amount of advertising that comes from the probiotic industry, you would think they do everything from regulating your GI system to keeping your vagina healthy to promoting world peace. Once again, we need to look at what actually has science behind it before we jump on the probiotic bandwagon.

PROBIOTIC

a microorganism that, when taken in large enough doses, can help the host (that is, you!). These are considered the "good" strains of bacteria and yeast that, when taken, can help with certain medical issues or treat certain conditions.

We've been told probiotics:
- Balance vaginal pH
- Treat frequent vaginal infections
- Combat antibiotics that might kill off the good vaginal bacteria
- Prevent recurrent bladder infections

These all sound like really good things, right? I would be all for them, too, if we had the evidence that probiotics actually helped accomplish any of them. Yes, there is evidence to support the use of probiotics for issues like antibiotic-associated diarrhea and infant colic, to name a few, but when it comes to the vagina, the evidence just isn't there yet.

The studies we *do* have are small and, for the most part, not up to scientific standards. This means probiotics *may* work as they're marketed to, but we just haven't proven it yet.

In addition, when supplements are analyzed in independent labs, there is often a discrepancy between what the bottle claims the supplement contains and what is actually there. That is, the dose may vary (sometimes even from pill to pill!), or the actual supplement listed as the primary ingredient is not what is in the pills, or they contain additional ingredients that are not declared on the label. This might sound surprising, but, frankly, to me—as a doctor—it isn't. This is what happens when an industry is largely unregulated: Probiotics sold as dietary supplements in the U.S. don't require approval by the FDA.

When it comes to vaginal probiotics, these supplements can take the form of pills, powders, and suppositories to place in the vagina. If you've read this far, you know how I feel about sticking things in your vagina—there has to be a good reason for it! It shouldn't just be because someone who wants to make a profit is trying to convince you that you need their product to achieve vaginal nirvana.

My one caveat: If you are someone who has struggled with diagnostically proven infections and your doctor recommends vaginal probiotics, these potentially can help when other treatments have been exhausted. If going this route, use the strain of probiotic your doctor recommends and be sure there is a long-term monitoring and follow-up plan.

The takeaways on why I would skip these products unless they are directly recommended by your doctor:

- There is a lack of scientific proof that they work.
- They can be rather expensive.
- They can mess with your natural vaginal ecosystem (remember, these are living microorganisms).
- In continuing to give these companies your money, you send the message to the industry that you are OK with the scant studies they have. Use your purchasing power and demand better science!

Can I pop the bumps
down there?

If you're like me, watching medical shows where things get popped is a perverse form of enjoyment, and you just can't look away. But I am here to ask you to please resist the urge to pop anything down there.

If you've got a bump in your pubic area, it could be a few things: an ingrown hair, cyst, abscess, STI . . . a lot of different possibilities!

Most of the time when I get this question, however, it's an ingrown hair, so I am going to focus on that.

> **INGROWN HAIR**
>
> when a hair gets trapped underneath the skin, or it exits the skin but then curls back and the end gets buried back into the skin. It can lead to red, itchy bumps.

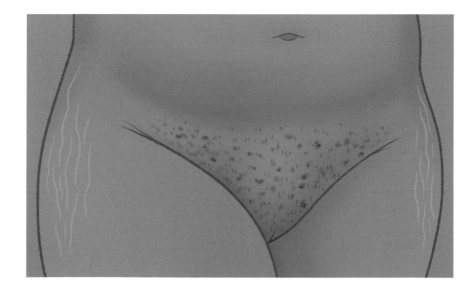

The temptation to pop these is real! However, doing so can cause more skin trauma and let in bacteria that can lead to an infection. Popping can lead to a collection of pus called an abscess or a skin infection caused cellulitis, both of which are way worse than the ingrown hair you started with!

So, what's a person to do when they've got one (or many) of these? I recommend trying the following:

1. Do nothing. Most go away on their own.
2. If you want to do something, apply a warm, wet washcloth to the area a few times a day. That can help work the hair out.
3. Do not under any circumstance go digging to get the hair out if it isn't already poking out.
4. If it is, use something like sterile tweezers (you can sterilize in boiling water or rubbing alcohol) to gently pluck out the hair. If it doesn't come easily, stop!

See your doctor if it's getting bigger, causing a lot of pain, getting red or pus-filled, or bothering you—they can try to remove it or prescribe some medication to help.

How do I know if my
labia are normal?

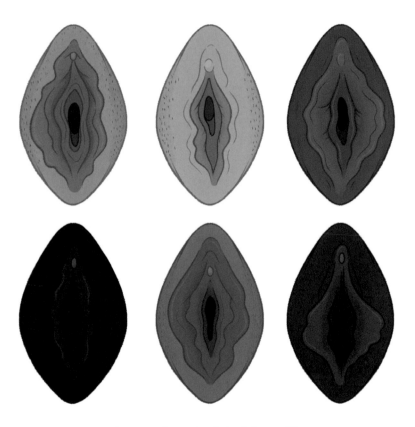

Just a small sample of what's "normal."

No two labia are the same! They come in all different shapes, skin tones, and sizes. Variations are even normal on the same person, with two sides rarely being identical!

LABIA

the lips of the vulva comprise two parts, inner (labia minora) and outer (labia majora).

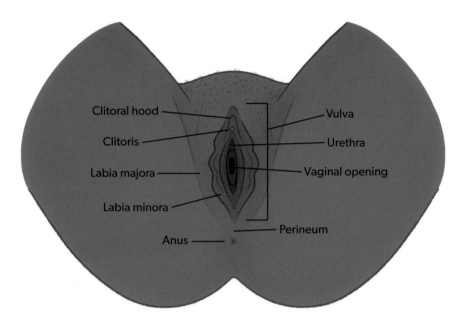

Variety is the spice of life, and here Mother Nature makes no exception. Why, then, do some people feel ashamed when their inner labia are longer than their outer lips or when one side is longer than the other? Why do they feel the need to have surgery to make their labia look more like what is often seen in the porn industry?

I have gotten so many messages from followers about the way their labia look, worried that something is wrong and needs to be fixed.

Here is how I respond when I am asked if your labia are normal: Yes, they are.

- Some labia are long.
- Some are short.
- Some are tucked in.
- Others protrude out.
- Some are uneven.
- Some are darker than the surrounding skin.

Seeing is believing, and since it's probably a little awkward to ask to see someone else's labia, this resource is my absolute go-to: The Labia Library (http://www.labialibrary.org.au/). Here you'll find a collection of photographs of different labia, showing just how unique each labia is.

If your labia have new growths, suddenly change in size, make activities like exercise or sex uncomfortable, or make you worried enough that something is wrong, of course seeing your doctor is a good idea. But luckily, the great majority of labia are just like you—unique, beautiful, and perfect just as they are.

Can I lighten
my labia?

This one makes me sad.

The world has taught us that lighter skin is better and darker skin is bad. We've been propagating this harmful, racist idea for centuries, and our ideas about the vulva haven't escaped such misinformed prejudice.

Can you lighten your labia? Sure. Spend time on Google and you'll find creams and gels that exist just for this purpose. There are also "cosmetic gynecologists" who can combine these with laser light treatments.

Just what your vulva never knew it needed . . .

. . . because it doesn't.

The skin of your vulva is often darker than skin elsewhere on your body, and that is *normal*. It happens because during puberty your hormone levels change, and this can lead to a darkening of the labia. Some women have darker ones than others. Again, this is perfectly normal.

If you're worried about *new* skin changes, please let your doctor know so she can make sure you aren't dealing with something more serious. But if your labia have always looked a certain way and you're just feeling self-conscious, please don't turn to treatments that only exist to capitalize on your insecurities.

POSSIBLE SIDE EFFECTS OF VAGINAL LIGHTENING:			
Empty wallet $$$	Allergic reaction	Swelling	Redness
Blistering	Irritation	Burning	Scarring

Can I ask my doctor to
shorten my labia?

Yes, you *can*, but I strongly encourage you to think twice about doing so.

> **LABIAPLASTY**
> the surgical term for surgically changing the appearance
> of the labia, either the inner (minora) or outer (majora) lips.
> Usually, they are made smaller by tissue removal for aesthetic
> reasons.

Who performs these surgeries? It's a wide cast of characters including
OB-GYNs, cosmetic surgeons, and plastic surgeons. As you can imagine,
experience and training varies greatly from surgeon to surgeon.

So back to your question—yes, you can ask your doctor to perform this
surgery. But I would want you to consider your motivation first. Has someone
made you feel ugly or imperfect? Has a partner told you that your labia are
abnormal? If so, that is not OK, and I beg you to reconsider (and give those
people the boot from your life).

There are some situations where surgery might be medically indicated
(and covered by insurance when otherwise it is often not). For example: labia
that are long enough that they are causing extreme pain during sex or physical
activity. But that's fairly uncommon.

What I'm talking about is cosmetic surgery; that is, surgery that does not
have a medical need. When it comes to your labia, it is really important to think
before you proceed with this kind of intervention. Risks of surgery can include:

- Surgical site infection
- Scarring
- Loss of sensation (the labia play a big role in sexual sensation!)
- Chronic nerve pain leading to pelvic pain or pain with sex

- Wound separation
- Need for repeat surgeries

If you do go down this road, be *very picky* about whom you choose as a surgeon. Don't be shy asking about training (did they do a weekend genital cosmetic procedure course or a yearslong residency?) and surgical volume (do they perform a handful of cases a year or many more than that?).

Closing statement: Current data shows that genital cosmetic surgery does *not* improve body image, sex drive, or satisfaction with sex. Be sure to stop and reflect on that before deciding whether or not you need this procedure.

How do I
tighten my vagina?

If you've read this far, you know what I'm going to ask: Why do you think you need to tighten it?

It is true that you can find lots of advertisements for procedures that can "tighten your vagina," and that in doing so you can increase your sexual satisfaction. Get your sensation back. Rekindle that spark in the bedroom.

Unfortunately, there is so much wrong with these claims . . . so let's dive in:

1. The vagina is a tube that is meant to dilate; for example, to let in a penis or let out a baby. It does not stay dilated forever and is perfectly capable of returning to its normal capacity after sex and childbirth.

2. The great majority of people with vaginas orgasm from clitoral stimulation and not vaginal penetration. So, I wonder whom the vaginal rejuvenating is really for.

3. The idea behind these procedures puts the thrust of sexual satisfaction on the vagina, when we know that *the brain* is the most important organ when it comes to arousal and sexual satisfaction.

So, what are these procedures exactly? In general, they are the same surgeries that we use to treat prolapse issues. That is, if the uterus, bladder, vagina, or rectum are unable to be properly supported by the pelvic tissue and muscles, we can surgically add additional support.

Yes, sometimes pelvic organ prolapse causes issues with sex, but that's not always the case. Meaning: A prolapse surgery is not always needed for sexual issues, and rebranding these surgeries as "vaginal rejuvenation" is false advertising. The type of pelvic reconstructive surgeries for prolapse are procedures that fix true anatomic abnormalities, and what people are passing off as surgeries for rejuvenation are not comparable.

Other procedures claim that using lasers or radiofrequency will tighten the vagina. In 2018, the FDA issued a statement that none of these devices were approved for the use of cosmetic vaginal surgery. Side effects can include burns, scarring, and pain during sex.

Bottom line: If sex is an issue, this is *definitely* something to dive into with your OB-GYN. We can do an exam and see if there are physical issues we can address, and if not, we can go deeper and explore whether something like referral to a sex therapist might be helpful.

Is it normal to
leak urine sometimes?

I want to address this because urinary leakage can be a taboo topic. Lots of people experience it, but few want to discuss it. It can feel really embarrassing, especially if you are young and you think the only people who are supposed to pee their pants are toddlers and old people in nursing homes.

So, once again, in the spirit of combatting the shame, let's get it out in the open.

Leaking urine, also known as urinary incontinence, is common. It affects approximately 25 percent of young women and up to 57 percent of middle-aged and postmenopausal women. That means that if you are leaking urine, you are most certainly not alone.

Not all urine leakage is the same. Here are some different types:

STRESS INCONTINENCE
leakage with laughing, jumping, coughing, sneezing

URGENCY INCONTINENCE
the "gotta-go-RIGHT-now-oops-I-peed-on-the-way" kind of leakage

MIXED INCONTINENCE
a combo of both above

COITAL INCONTINENCE
leakage during sex

NOCTURNAL ENURESIS
peeing the bed at night

Other types exist, too, but these are the kind we commonly see.

There is no need to suffer in silence. If you've stopped exercising, stopped having sex, or no longer take long road trips because you are leaking or can't make it to the bathroom in time, please let your doctor know.

They can ask some questions and do an exam, rule out causes like infection, and potentially send you to a specialist for further evaluation. Treatments depend on the cause and may include medication, surgical procedures, lifestyle modifications, pelvic floor therapy, or a combination of the above.

Don't be ashamed to discuss this with your gynecologist! I promise you that we have heard it all and have probably even been peed on when evaluating patients. It's no big deal for a doctor—just another day at the office.

CHAPTER 3

Facts for Feeling Good

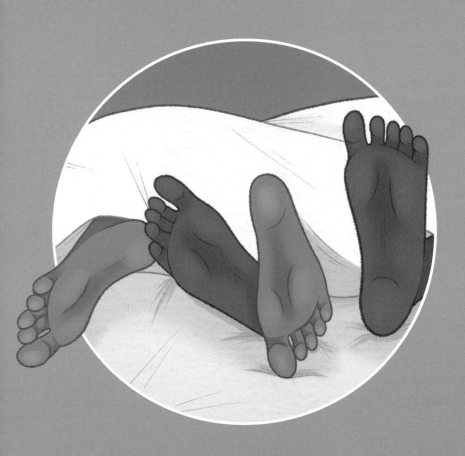

If I masturbate too much, is that bad?

Masturbation is something I was never taught about in school, other than that it was not a holy endeavor and should be avoided. Thanks, Sister Claire.

Masturbating should only be qualified as "too much" if it's doing any of the following:

- Getting in the way of your normal activities
- Causing physical symptoms that are painful or uncomfortable (think chafing)
- Causing relationship problems
- Causing *you* distress

Really, that's it. And you can see how this is, for the most part, subjective and will vary from person to person.

Masturbation can be a really important part of your sexuality. Little kids naturally do it as a way of exploring their bodies and because it just feels good. Masturbating can show you what you like, which, in turn, you can show your partner for a more fulfilling sexual relationship. It gives you the power of being in charge of your pleasure and not relying on someone else. And it can be a great way to relieve stress.

All the myths about masturbation—you'll go blind, you'll become infertile, your nerves will be damaged, you'll become homosexual (seriously?!), it means your marriage is not fulfilling, it will stunt your emotional development or give you cancer—are all just that: myths.

These falsehoods likely persisted through the ages as the result of poor education and the fear that masturbating teens will become sex-obsessed fiends who won't ever leave their bedrooms. It's just not true—discovering masturbation is a totally normal and healthy part of sexual development.

If you are worried that you are doing it too much and it is interfering with school, work, or your relationship (because your partner feels you prioritize it over them, for example), let your doctor know. We can review strategies and help point you in the right direction.

If sex and putting in tampons hurt, what do I do?

Here's what I *don't* want you to do: grin and bear it and think this is just how life is.

The feeling that your muscles are clenched too tight or that you or your partner are physically hitting a wall could be signs of vaginismus.

VAGINISMUS

when the muscles of the vaginal opening involuntarily spasm or are excessively tight, making things like having sex, inserting a tampon, or having a pelvic exam painful and/or difficult.

Vaginismus is a true medical condition and not something that is "all in your head" and that you can just wish away. It can develop as the result of:

- Prior sexual or physical trauma
- Difficult childbirth
- Prior pelvic surgeries
- Anxiety
- Fear of sex
- Vulvar nerve and skin conditions
- Chronic pain elsewhere such as pelvic or abdominal pain

Your doctor can diagnose it based on what you tell her and what she sees on physical exam. She will likely try to insert a finger and/or speculum as well as assess the level of contraction on your pelvic muscles when she examines you.

Keep in mind this is not something you consciously do like contracting your bicep muscle—that is easy to tighten and relax, right? This is when your pelvic floor muscles are involuntarily contracting or staying in a state of sustained contraction all the time. Ouch!

The good news: You don't have to live with this forever. Treatments exist and with them many patients get relief. Your doctor may recommend a combination of:

- Pelvic floor physical therapy
- Sex or cognitive-based therapy
- Topical lubricants, moisturizers, or numbing creams
- Vaginal dilators (think starting really small and working your way up—this can be done solo or with the guidance of a physical therapist)

How do I
clean a dildo?

Excellent question because cleaning them after every use is important!

You should clean sex toys after each use and before sharing them with a partner.

However, cleaning and disinfecting doesn't protect against everything. That's why even though we are taught sharing is caring, it really isn't with these kinds of toys. But if you must, using a new condom each time can make it a little safer.

That said, let's break down cleaning and disinfecting. What you can and can't use varies by the type of toy and the material.

THINGS THAT CAN SPREAD ON SEX TOYS:

- HPV
- Scabies
- Gonorrhea
- Chlamydia
- . . . and more!

	CLEANING	DISINFECTING
What it is	Removes discharge and debris	Goal is to remove bacteria and viruses that can infect you
How to	Use soap and warm water either with a washcloth or by submerging.	1. Submerge in 0.5% bleach for 3 minutes or 70% isopropyl alcohol for 5 minutes. 2. Wash afterward with soap and water. 3. If silicone or stainless steel, you can boil or use the dishwasher sanitizer mode.
Cautions	• Avoid soap with fragrances—use the same kinds recommended for your vulva! • Remove batteries.	• If the material is porous (i.e., rubber, latex, PVC), then you cannot disinfect. • We aren't sure if the alcohol method kills certain viruses like HPV. • UV light sterilization devices are out there but not well regulated. • Remove batteries (bears repeating!). • Don't boil or put anything with batteries in the dishwasher.
Disclaimer	Always check your product's instructions to see what is recommended and what isn't!	

What lubes are
OK to use?

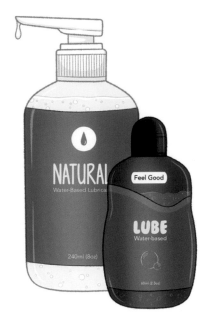

Bravo to you for asking this question and realizing that lube is not just for people who've gone through menopause. I applaud you!

Lube is awesome. It can make sex more exciting, the use of toys easier, and even help with masturbation. What's not to love?

Not all lubes are created equal, though, so you need to pick the one that's right for you and your sexual circumstances.

No matter which one you pick, avoid fragrances and scents—they can cause nasty irritation to your vulva. Chemicals like parabens and phthalates are also a no go, since they are endocrine disruptors (chemicals that interfere with our hormones) and can be cancer causing.

Water-based: gentle on the skin but can dry quickly. Not great in the shower, as it washes away.
Example: ASTROGLIDE, pjur AQUA

Silicone-based: very silky and lasts a long time but hard to wash off and shouldn't be used with sex toys or diaphragms.
Example: Überlube

Oil-based: like silicone but also can be used as a massage oil. Causes condoms to break, so do not use it if you rely on them for birth control or STI prevention! Also can be hard to wash off and can stain sheets.
Example: coconut oil

Check out the diagram below to pick the one that might work best for you!

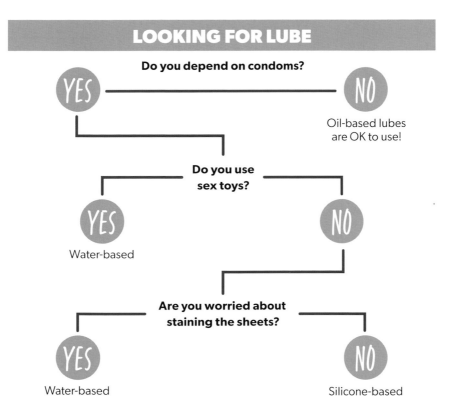

LOOKING FOR LUBE

Do you depend on condoms?

YES — NO

Oil-based lubes
are OK to use!

**Do you use
sex toys?**

YES   NO

Water-based

**Are you worried about
staining the sheets?**

YES   NO

Water-based   Silicone-based

Where is my
G-spot?

Ah, the G-spot. Like Bigfoot and the lost city of Atlantis, it is rumored to exist . . . yet there's no agreement if it's real, and it often involves a lot of searching and frustration.

The G-spot, aka the Gräfenberg spot (named for the German physician who first described it in the medical literature in 1950), is alleged to be a specialized erotic zone located in the vagina that, when stimulated, provides significant pleasure.

It's supposed to be located on the front wall of the vagina just under the urethra (the hole where urine comes out), about a third of the way in.

There is significant disagreement in the medical community about whether it exists: Some swear it does, while others point to lack of scientific evidence. A review in 2012 looked at studies from 1950 to 2011 to see if any objective data existed to prove the existence of the G-spot, and they concluded that while the majority of women believes it exists, there is no strong or consistent evidence to prove that is so.

Does it really matter if there's a specific anatomic structure with a designated name if being stimulated there feels good? I say no—do what works for you!

However, this matters when unscrupulous people try to make money by selling something called a "G-shot" or "O-shot" to allegedly pump up your sex life. These are injections of platelet-rich plasma (PRP) or collagen that are supposed to bulk up your G-spot.

There is *no data* these work, and they could lead to injury or infection. Best-case scenario, you leave with an empty wallet and likely no improvement in your sex life, when more evidence-based therapy and treatment could have been a much better investment.

Will I bleed the
first time I have sex?

Maybe, maybe not.

There seems to be a lot wrapped up in the first time and whether or not you bleed. If you don't, does it mean you lied and weren't really a virgin? Or should you prepare with multiple sheets and towels because it might look like a crime scene after you're done?

It can be an extra layer of worry when you might already be a little nervous about what your first time is like.

Yes, bleeding the first time you have sex is totally possible. Most commonly, it happens when the hymen tears a bit and there's some bleeding from those torn edges. Usually, it's just a bit, and there's nothing you need to do about it—it stops on its own. Why people refer to this as "cherry popping" is something I will never understand.

Lack of bleeding is perfectly normal, too, however. Some people have already used tampons, dildos, or inserted their fingers, and their hymens have already stretched or torn. For others, it happens because of physical activity not related to sex. And still others just don't have any hymenal tearing because of how their hymen is naturally shaped. Hymens come in different shapes—just like everything in nature, really. Check out examples of some on the next page.

Bleeding can come from other things, too, so it's important to keep that in mind. Some of those things could be:

- Lack of lubrication leading to lacerations
- Blood vessels on the outside of the cervix that are delicate sometimes bleed (often nothing to be concerned about)
- Rough sex causing lacerations
- Infections like STIs
- Cancer (this is RARE!)

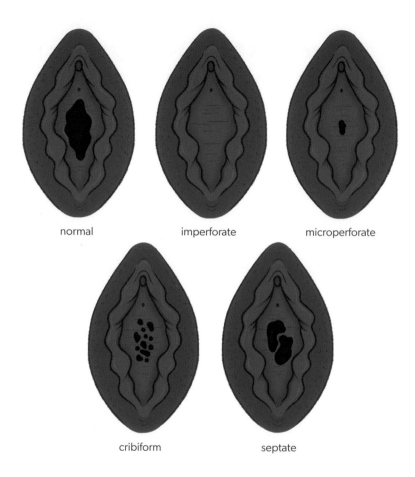

normal   imperforate   microperforate

cribiform   septate

If you bleed a lot—like you are soaking pads or towels and it isn't stopping—you should definitely seek care right away. Otherwise, know that bleeding a little after your first time is not something to worry about.

My partner says they won't go down on me unless I wax all my hair.
Should I do it?

As I've discussed on page 45, grooming your pubic hair is a personal choice. It offers no medical benefit, and pubic hair actually has a job to do.

If you want to remove it, that is your decision, and you can check out pages 46–47, where I describe ways to make hair removal safer and less prone to things like injury or infection.

However, if your partner makes you feel that you *need* to remove some or all of your pubic hair in order for them to perform certain sexual acts with you, that's a separate issue. Answering these questions might be illuminating when deciding how to respond:

- How do you feel about their suggestion?
- Did they make you feel embarrassed about your current grooming practices?
- Do they refer to your natural state as gross or undesirable?
- Do you feel that they are respecting your body?

If any of those answers leave you feeling ashamed, embarrassed, dirty, or weird, then I think you've got some bigger issues than your pubic hair. It may be that the person you are with doesn't appreciate you for you and has unrealistic ideas about what is normal thanks to the porn industry and societal pressure.

On the other hand, if your partner were engaging in this discussion respectfully and thought that hair removal could be a new experience that could enhance *your* pleasure or be a fun way for you to engage in some mutual fantasies, maybe it's something you might be interested in trying.

As always, it is your body and your choice. Do not ever let anyone shame you into how you handle your body or hold sexual experiences hostage in return for dictating your appearance.

Do over-the-counter
libido supplements really work?

There is no shortage of pills being marketed to women as libido enhancers, and this market is only growing. Often these pills contain a blend of "natural" supplements that claim to:

- Induce relaxation
- Enhance enjoyment
- Support desire
- Improve your orgasms
- Boost your energy

It all sounds great, right?

Here's the thing: We have little to no quality data that these supplements work. They are not regulated by the FDA so it is hard to know what is actually in each pill or if other undeclared ingredients are present. But what is most concerning is that these supplements can cause very real side effects. Issues like hallucinations, anxiety, insomnia, chest pain, high blood pressure, and more have been reported.

At the center of the appeal of these supplements is the libido, which is complex—it's highly personal and not just an on or off switch that a pill can address. Issues with arousal, orgasm, and sexual dysfunction are very real. In fact, they affect about 43 percent of American women, with 12 percent saying it causes them personal distress.

These people deserve real evaluation and treatment—not products that prey on insecurities with unproven efficacy and lots of possible side effects.

If you are struggling with low libido, know that your doctor can help get to the root of the problem and can counsel you on evidence-based treatments like sex therapy, couples therapy, physical therapy, or medications that have more data than what you might find online or in the supplement aisle of your grocery store.

Is anal sex
bad for me?

Anal sex is not uncommon: 10 percent of teens report having tried it and 36 to 44 percent of adults aged 25–44 have too. And with the right precautions, anal sex can be part of a healthy sex life without any harm.

The anus and rectum do not make lubrication in the same way the vagina does, so it is important to use plenty of lube. Using lube (see page 70 for my advice on this), going slowly, and stopping if something hurts are important to making sure you don't cause any tears, which you really want to avoid. If those do occur, they are more likely to get infected, given what is in the intestines— lots of bacteria and fecal material—so don't be afraid to speak up to your partner if something doesn't feel right.

Anal sex also has a higher risk of spreading STIs, especially HIV, but, again, you can use some common sense to decrease your risk. Use condoms, get tested, and don't share sex toys. Keep in mind that oral infections such as herpes can spread to the anus if oral sex is involved.

If going from anal to vaginal sex, washing in between is a great idea to keep bacteria from transferring into the vagina. Use a new condom too!

Anal sex can potentially worsen existing hemorrhoids. Using lubrication can help, but if they are persistent or bothersome you can consider having them removed by a doctor.

Currently, there isn't good data to show that anal sex leads to stool leakage, also known as fecal incontinence. While one study did find this, its conclusions have not been widely accepted as other factors may have been the cause.

This might seem like a long list of things to keep in mind, but if anal sex is something you and your partner enjoy, these precautions will become easier with practice and will make the experience safer and more enjoyable for you.

What counts as
losing your virginity?

Virginity is a made-up contrivance.

You might have a hard time buying that, but ask yourself what "counts" when it comes to losing your virginity.

If we go by the more mainstream view of penis-in-vagina definition, that leaves out an entire population of people who never have that kind of sex. So, women who have sex with women: Are they virgins forever?

What about people who have anal sex? Oral sex?

It's not as straightforward as you think.

Virginity is a social construct—historically made up to cast virginal women as desirable and reinforce the patriarchal control that requiring a woman be "pure" for her future husband implies.

You get to decide your definition of virginity, and I don't get to tell you whether it's right or wrong—and neither does anyone else.

CHAPTER 4

Itching and Burning

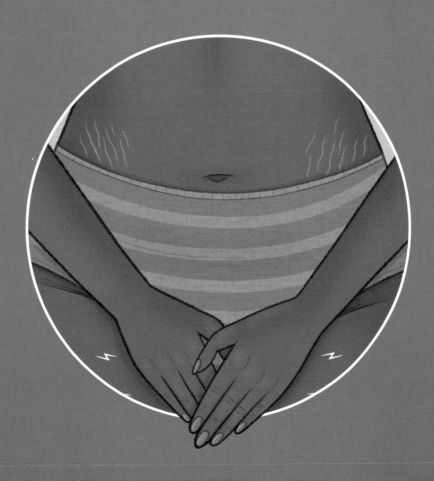

Is it OK to use drugstore medicines to treat my yeast infection?

Before I answer that, I've got a question for you: How do you know you have a yeast infection?

The truth is, the symptom we typically think of as indicating a yeast infection—thick, white, cottage-cheese discharge—doesn't always correlate with an actual yeast infection.

What that means: Just because you *think* you have a yeast infection doesn't mean you do (especially if it's your first).

Because of this, I recommend skipping the self-diagnosis and seeing your doctor if you have concerns about discharge or vaginal complaints. When face-to-face, we can take a good history, do a thorough exam, and do some basic diagnostic testing. Then, if we have confirmed yeast, you have my blessing to use the OTC yeast medications or use one prescribed by me.

"But that is such a waste of time and money!!" is something you might be thinking right now. I get it. But when people with vaginas self-diagnose, many do so incorrectly. This leads to money wasted, time wasted, and a delay in treating something else that might become more complicated—and more difficult to treat.

Even the drug companies who make these yeast medicines agree. For example, on the box of Monistat you will see the following: "Do not use if you have never had a vaginal yeast infection diagnosed by a doctor." Give us a call before you buy!

Should I avoid sugar if I'm
prone to yeast infections?

If you google (and we all do), you'll see lots of recommendations for preventing yeast infections, especially if you are someone who gets them a lot.

There is even a diet called the "candida diet" that claims to reduce yeast infections (among other things) if followed. If you follow this diet, you are told to take probiotics and avoid:

- Simple sugars (including many fruits)
- Rice
- White flour
- Gluten
- Whole milk
- Cheese
- Ketchup
- Foods containing yeast
- Beer, wine, and liquor
- Coffee and tea (considered "optional" . . . how kind)

That isn't even the entire list.

So, to recap: No grain. No sugar. No CHEESE.

For most people, that's not a fun way to live. If you are asking someone to follow this strict diet, then there had better be some good data showing it is worth it and it works, right?

And yet, there isn't.

To date, there is no good evidence that this diet is protective against vulvovaginal yeast infections. There just isn't. If that doesn't make you mad (may I repeat: NO CHEESE), then I don't know what will.

But let's step back and just think about sugar. I think some of the confusion that sugar makes you prone to yeast infections is the fact that diabetics are more prone to these infections. The logical jump to increased sugar being the cause of these infections is easy to make, but even if you eat a ton of sugar in one sitting, unless you're diabetic, your body is able to process it.

Another example of why this diet doesn't make sense: the recommendation to avoid foods with yeast. The yeast that causes the majority of vaginal yeast infections is *Candida albicans*, and the yeast found in most breads and fermented goods is *Saccharomyces cerevisiae*. All yeast is not the same, so this is another big red flag that we're not dealing with good science.

Listen, if you want to avoid some of these foods for lifestyle reasons, I don't have a problem with that. But don't be fooled into thinking it will solve your yeast woes.

Consider this permission to have the cheese.

Why do my
yeast infections keep coming back?

These suck—I'm sorry.

First, let's define what these even are.

> **RECURRENT YEAST INFECTIONS**
>
> four or more separate infections in 12 months.

As I mentioned on page 80, self-diagnosis doesn't always get it right, and many infections that are thought to be yeast infections aren't at all.

This means in order to carry an accurate diagnosis of recurrent yeast infections, you should have four *documented* diagnoses. And the best test for this includes a yeast culture, which is when your doctor sends a swab to the lab and, rather than getting just a yes/no answer about the presence of yeast, the lab puts it in culture, lets it grow, and is able to determine the exact strain of yeast you have. This is ideal, since many people with vaginas who have recurrent infections have some less-common strains that are not cured with traditional medications.

OK, now that we know what it is and how we diagnose it, how do we make them stop?!

Treatment is often two pronged:

Acute therapy: daily antifungal treatment for an extended period of time
Suppression therapy: usually, weekly oral or vaginal antifungal treatment, sometimes done for months at a time

Most people on this regimen get long-term cure and relief. However, close monitoring during this time is important, because if you aren't getting better, your doctor needs to know. Sometimes referral to a vulvovaginal specialist is needed for the really tough cases, so don't hesitate to bring that up with your doctor.

Certain things can make you prone to yeast infections, such as diabetes, recent antibiotic use, immunosuppression, and possibly as a side effect of some birth control pills. The last one is potentially due to higher estrogen levels helping yeast to grow and stick to vaginal cells.

So, what *can* you do other than taking antifungal medication to prevent recurrent yeast infections? These are the evidence-based interventions that can help:

- Avoid douches
- Avoid feminine hygiene washes
- Wear breathable underwear
- Change out of wet clothes

What about the "candida diet" for recurrent infections? I've already discussed why that's not helpful on pages 81–82, so be sure to read up on that, since many women think they need it if they are prone to recurrent infections. And if you're curious about the role of boric acid suppositories in treating tough yeast cases, that just happens to be coming up next.

Boric acid suppositories—
do they work?

They can definitely be useful for treating certain infections, but that doesn't mean you should run out and buy a bottle to keep in your medicine cabinet. Let's talk why.

It seems boric acid suppositories can be found everywhere these days: in the supplement section of drugstores, from online wellness brands that "promote" vaginal health, and on social media where (often paid) users swear by them.

Proposed benefits of boric acid suppositories include:
- pH regulation
- "supporting" the vaginal environment
- elimination of odors
- treatment of infections

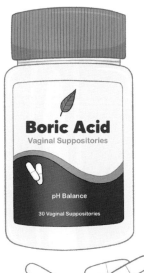

. . . all while being over the counter and supposedly safe to use for 7–14 day courses, or after you have sex, or after your period, or whenever things seem off.

That seems pretty broad and without a lot of clear guidance, don't you think?

My main concern with all supplements is that they're often used by those who are self-treating without an actual diagnosis. They then may delay care and, when they are finally seen, end up having a bigger problem than when they started.

These suppositories can also be **fatal if ingested,** and I worry about them being kept casually in medicine cabinets. Heck, I've had followers message me on social media telling me they didn't realize they were for vaginal use and not a pill to be swallowed until after the fact! Yikes!!

The heart of what bothers me is that companies that promote these suppositories make it sound like the vagina is something that needs constant monitoring and balancing, and it really doesn't. Vaginas usually work pretty well on their own, and when they don't, your health care team should weigh in.

Now that I've said all that, I *will* say that sometimes boric acid suppositories are useful. As physicians, we sometimes recommend them for people who have recurrent yeast or bacterial vaginosis infections, or resistant trichomonas infections.

In fact, we have regimens that we can follow when it comes to using boric acid. That means we have certain lengths of times we recommend use, often coupled with vaginal or oral antibiotics. It's very different from just occasionally using one when you feel things are "off" down there.

My take-home message is this: Boric acid suppositories *do* have a role in treating certain infections. However, they should not by any means be thought of as a cure-all that anyone can just pop in whenever they think their vagina needs some freshening up.

Remember, the supplement industry has a stake in making you feel you need to constantly do something to keep your delicate flower balanced. Don't play into their hands—you are smarter than that!

Will garlic cure a
yeast infection?

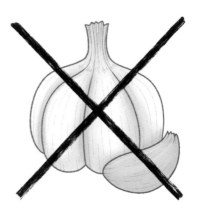

Garlic is meant for things like pasta sauce and garlic bread—not your vagina!

This is another all-natural trend that has become widely popular. Supporters of turning your vagina into salad dressing claim that garlic contains a compound that has been shown to kill yeast in a lab. Sure, that may be true—but this is where an understanding of science is important. What happens in a lab and what happens in a vagina are two very different things.

In fact, studies published so far have not shown *any* effect when garlic was used vaginally.

Is it so bad to try if you're suffering at home and want to just try something, *anything*? I say yes. Putting food in your vagina is just a bad idea. Bacteria can be present that can then be introduced into your body. The mucosal lining of the vagina is sensitive and adding in foreign bodies can throw off your pH and lead to a worsening of your symptoms. And maybe most importantly—trying to self-treat with completely non-evidence-based therapies is a poor substitute for having your medical issues seen, heard, and taken seriously.

Yes to garlic in pesto.

No to garlic in private parts.

Is bacterial vaginosis an STI?

No—in fact, it's not a true infection at all.

BACTERIAL VAGINOSIS (BV)

a clinical condition caused by an overgrowth of a certain kind of bacteria in the vagina with an undergrowth of the good bacteria, lactobacilli. Think of it as an out-of-balance vaginal situation. It is the most common cause of abnormal vaginal discharge.

Gardnerella vaginalis, Bacteroides, Peptostreptococcus, Fusobacterium, Prevotella, Atopobium vaginae

Lactobacilli

BV is not a specific bacteria that is spread during sex, but it *is* found more commonly in sexually active women. Having a new sex partner or multiple sex partners can be a risk factor, though we don't exactly know why.

Other things can make having BV more likely, too, such as douching, or inserting other products in the vagina (rinses, washes, yoni pearls).

The typical BV discharge is thin and gray, fishy, and may cause burning or itching in the vagina or on the vulva. BV is treated with antibiotics that you take by mouth or place in the vagina.

Having trouble with BV that just doesn't seem to quit? I've got you covered in the next question.

My BV infections won't go away—
what do I do?

Bacterial vaginosis (BV) can be really annoying, especially if it seems like it never goes away or keeps coming back. Check out page 88, where I talk about what BV is (and isn't).

First things first: Confirm your diagnosis (am I a broken record yet?!). Resist the urge to self-diagnose and see your doctor so you can know exactly what is going on.

Types of BV infections:

RECURRENT BV
three separate documented infections in 12 months.

RESISTANT BV
does not go away after prescribed treatment.

It's important to let your doctor know if your symptoms don't go away or if you think they've returned so that an accurate diagnosis can be made, and then they can help you with a good, evidence-based treatment plan.

Options for resistant or recurrent BV include:

- A repeat dose of the same antibiotics (oral or vaginal)
- A different kind of antibiotic (oral or vaginal)
- Suppressive antibiotic therapy used twice weekly or monthly for up to six months to keep infections from returning
- A combination of oral antibiotics followed by boric acid suppositories (see page 85 for more on that) followed by suppressive therapy (whew!)
- Referral to an infectious disease or vulvovaginal specialist

- Vaginal probiotics. (See page 49, where I cover that in more detail. Keep in mind data on probiotics for vaginal health is limited, it is important to use the correct strain of probiotic, and you should discuss usage with your doctor so you have a good plan in place to monitor if they are helping or not.)

Sexual partners do *not* need to be treated, as BV is not thought to be a sexually transmitted infection. However, don't forget that certain things can make you more prone to BV, such as douching and feminine washes, so definitely stop using them if you are!

How do I know
if I have an STI?

STI

a sexually transmitted infection. The preferred term over sexually transmitted disease (STD), since not all infections cause disease and not all infections have symptoms.

Some symptoms of STIs include:

- Yellow, green, or frothy vaginal discharge
- Strong vaginal odor
- Having to pee more frequently
- Burning or stinging when you pee
- Bleeding in between periods
- Bleeding with sex
- Abdominal or pelvic pain
- Bleeding, discharge, itching, or pain in your rectum
- Bumps, sores, growths, or blisters near your mouth, genitals, or buttocks
- Burning, itching, or tingling in the genital area
- Yellowing skin (jaundice) with nausea, vomiting, fatigue, dark urine, and loss of appetite
- Fever, swollen lymph glands, rash, fatigue, weight loss, diarrhea

However, here's the thing: Many times—especially in those assigned female at birth—STIs aren't obvious. That means you can have one and not know it, so you can also spread it to partners unknowingly.

If you've never been tested, have a new partner, have symptoms, or just want peace of mind, ask your doctor to be screened (and see page 92, where I talk about what is commonly screened for at these visits). You're definitely earning your adult card when you do.

When I ask for STI testing, what does my doctor order?

STI testing is not a single order or batch of tests that are done the same way for every person, everywhere. This is why it is *really* important to know what you have—and haven't!—been tested for.

In general (but clarify with *your* doctor about what they ordered for *you*), STI testing at a minimum includes screening for:
- Gonorrhea
- Chlamydia
- HIV
- Syphilis
- HPV (usually not done until age 30 given current guidelines, as it often clears prior to this)

Additional tests you may be screened for (or may wish to request):
- Trichomoniasis
- Hepatitis B and C
- Herpes

I want to dive into herpes more because it's important to understand how screening can be confusing. If you don't have any lesions that might indicate herpes, then your doctor can screen for it by doing a blood test to look for antibodies. The test can tell if you have antibodies to either HSV types 1 or 2 (see page 97, where I discuss the differences between these strains), the presence of which mean you have been previously exposed.

However, it's important to note that these results can be hard to interpret. Antibody testing can't tell you:
- If you have oral or genital herpes definitively
- When you were exposed

Considering that HSV-1 is so common, screening might bring more distress than useful information. This is one reason why the United States Preventive Services Task Force does not recommend screening for people who have no symptoms concerning for herpes.

It's really important to be informed before you have any testing done, especially when it comes to herpes screening. Will the testing help or just add more confusion to your sex life? Have a conversation with your doctor so you understand what it is you're being screened for and what you might do with that information once you get your results.

I have chlamydia, but I don't want to tell my partner . . . .
Do I have to?

I understand that it can be awkward—and potentially relationship-ending to have these conversations—but I am going to ask that you do it.

If you don't, you're not doing anyone any favors. Not yourself (because if you get treatment and they don't, they will just pass it right back to you), not your partner (because their health can suffer if they don't get treated), and not society (this is how infections stick around).

If you need help having the conversation, you can ask your doctor. Many times I've discussed the infection with partners (with patient consent, of course!) either during a visit or over the phone.

In fact, I have often prescribed the antibiotics needed for STI treatment for male partners. Yes, me, an OB-GYN! And here's why: expedited partner therapy.

EXPEDITED PARTNER THERAPY

the practice of treating a partner for an STI without examining them or having them be your patient.

This means OB-GYNs can not only treat their patients with chlamydia or another infection but their partners too! It's perfectly legal, and the American College of Obstetricians and Gynecologists supports this. Why is this awesome? Because it means your partner doesn't have to set up an entirely separate visit with their own doctor—making it more likely they *will* get treated.

Listen, getting an STI sucks. But it's not uncommon, and it doesn't make you dirty or negligent. It makes you human. It may mean some uncomfortable conversations, but they are important to address head-on.

If someone doesn't want to be with you because of chlamydia, that might be something worth finding out sooner rather than later anyway, right?

Can lesbians
get STIs too?

Yes!

STIs can definitely spread between two assigned females at birth, including during oral sex, fingering, vulva-on-vulva contact, kissing, and sharing sex toys. This is why it's important to always be safe even if there isn't a penis involved.

Getting tested before anything goes down in the bedroom is always recommended, and repeat testing as needed if you are not in a mutually monogamous relationship.

Dental dams (a thin piece of latex or polyurethane plastic) can be used during oral sex to help decrease infection risk. You can use an actual dental dam or cut open a condom or latex glove. In a pinch, you can use plastic wrap, but keep in mind this hasn't been well studied. Whatever you use, use it once and throw it away—don't turn it over and use the other side or that defeats the purpose!

Latex gloves can help keep you safe during any practice where your fingers are inserted somewhere where bleeding might happen, such as the vagina or anus.

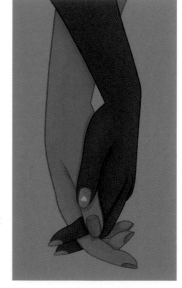

If you are using sex toys, see pages 68–69, where I talk about how to clean and disinfect them so you lower your chance of spreading infections. You can also use condoms on toys (and use a new one each time on each person), but the best thing to do is to not share at all and each have your own.

Lastly, don't forget about vaccinations that can protect against STIs such as the HPV and hepatitis B vaccines. Vaccines that prevent cancer are pretty awesome, if you ask me.

Do I have to tell my partner that
I get cold sores?

Ideally, yes.

Cold sores—aka fever blisters—are caused by the herpes virus. Most people are infected when they are children—it's *very* common! The virus can be spread to your partner, and that's why it's important to have an honest conversation about it.

Let's first review some quick facts about herpes, because there can be some confusion around this virus:

- There are two strains: herpes simplex type 1 (HSV-1) and herpes simplex type 2 (HSV-2).
- Oral herpes is *usually* from HSV-1.
- Genital herpes can be caused by *both* HSV-1 and HSV-2.
- Herpes is common! In the U.S., 48 percent of people have HSV-1, and 12 percent have HSV-2.
- An oral infection can become a genital infection from oral sex.

Herpes can spread even when you don't have an active outbreak, and this is another reason it's important to let your partner know if you have it. Think if the scenario were reversed and this information was withheld from you: How would that make you feel?

So it's important to disclose, and your partner should *not* shame you for having oral herpes—especially since it is so common as I mentioned earlier. If they do, you might want to reflect on that.

So what's a person to do if they've been diagnosed with oral herpes? Like I said, it can spread even when there are no obvious fever blisters, but the risk is much less likely then. Some ways to keep you and your partner safe include:

- Never share cups, straws, or utensils.
- Avoiding kissing or oral sex when you have a cold sore.
- If you start to feel a tingling or burning sensation near your mouth, that can be a sign of an impending outbreak—see above on what to avoid.

- Use condoms or dental dams (see page 96) to decrease the risk of spread during sexual contact.

Above all, please remember that cold sores are incredibly common and do *not* say anything about you as a person.

Can I contract an
infection just from oral sex?

Absolutely.
- HIV
- Herpes
- HPV
- Gonorrhea
- Chlamydia
- Syphilis
- Trichomoniasis
- Hepatitis

All of these can be spread from oral sex alone.

What's really concerning is how few people use protection (condoms and/or dental dams) during oral sex, likely because of the belief that oral sex is safer than vaginal sex. A survey of teens done in 2018 showed that only 8 percent and 9 percent of females and males used condoms during their most recent oral sex experience. Yikes!

These infections can be bad news. For example, HPV infections in the mouth and throat can lead to head and neck cancers, which are difficult and painful to treat, and since we don't routinely screen these areas for HPV, can be hard to diagnose.

Infections from common bacteria that live in the intestines can also spread during oral-anal sex, such as E.coli, Salmonella, Shigella, and even parasites like giardia.

Want to practice safe oral sex? Get tested regularly, and use barrier protection every time, especially if you are not in a monogamous relationship or you aren't sure of your partner's status. See page 96, where I discuss how to use a dental dam in case you're curious.

Which STIs are curable . . .
and which ones aren't?

Hearing you have an STI can be really life changing, and I don't think that is an exaggeration. Society has stigmatized STIs to the point where some people don't want to get tested out of fear, and others don't want to tell their partners their status because they feel ashamed.

Shame does no one any good—but education and information does.

Here's a review of which infections can be cured, which ones can't, and what that might mean:

	CURABLE?	COMMENTS
Gonorrhea	Yes	
Chlamydia	Yes	
Herpes simplex virus (HSV)	No	• Antiviral medication can treat outbreaks and help prevent recurrences. • Outbreaks tend to happen less frequently over time.
Human papillomavirus (HPV)	No	There's no cure, but HPV *may* clear on its own. We can't predict who will clear and who will go on to develop warts or cancer from different HPV strains—this is why vaccination and cervical cancer screening is key!

	CURABLE?	COMMENTS
Genital warts	No	• Treatments can help lessen the appearance or remove warts completely. These include topical medication, freezing, surgical removal. • Treatments do not completely eliminate the chances that the HPV virus that causes the warts will spread to sexual partners.
HIV	No	16% of HIV-positive adults in the U.S. don't know their HIV status! Get tested.
Syphilis	Yes	
Hepatitis	Sort of	• Some infections resolve on their own. • Immune globulin treatment can be used for some types.
Pelvic inflammatory disease (PID)	Yes	See pages 102–103 for more on PID.
Trichomoniasis	Yes	

It bears repeating: Sixteen percent of HIV-positive adults in the U.S. don't know their HIV status! Get tested.

When does chlamydia turn into PID
and cause infertility?

Pelvic inflammatory disease (PID) sounds scary, and I can understand why.

> **PELVIC INFLAMMATORY DISEASE**
> an inflammatory infection that happens when bacteria from the vagina move up to and infect the female reproductive organs. This includes the uterus (endometritis), fallopian tubes and ovaries (salpingitis and tubo-ovarian abscess), and the pelvic cavity (pelvic peritonitis).

Many of us were taught the damaging idea that if we have sex even once we will get chlamydia, which will morph into PID, which will mess up our fallopian tubes, and we will never be able to get pregnant, which is what we sexually active rule breakers deserve.

Luckily for everyone . . . it doesn't work like that.

PID affects about 1 million women in the United States every year—and that number may actually be higher, since many cases go undiagnosed.

We don't need to get into the weeds with diagnosis, but in order to be officially diagnosed with PID, you have to have a few of these findings:

- Fever
- Pain of the uterus/cervix/ovaries when touched on exam
- Abnormal cervical discharge
- Lab tests that are positive for gonorrhea or chlamydia

So, yes, chlamydia can cause PID—but it's not the only culprit. Other things that can lead to PID include gonorrhea as well as certain bacteria that may not have anything to do with sex, like bacteria normally found in the vagina but which can cause trouble when their growth goes unchecked. These include

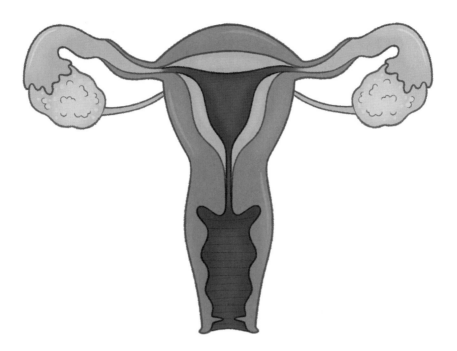

Gardnerella vaginalis and *Streptococcus agalactiae,* just to name a few. Newer data has shown that Mycoplasma, Ureaplasma, and some other less-common bacteria may also play a role in PID.

It's hard to say how long it takes PID to cause the scarring or damage to the fallopian tubes that might contribute to infertility. We just don't know, but certainly the longer it goes unchecked, the more likely this could be a consequence. However, it's important to note that some studies have shown that mild, even undetectable PID can also lead to higher infertility rates.

The bottom line? Seek care ASAP if you think you have a vaginal or pelvic infection. Don't delay getting diagnosed or treated, and make sure that if your partner is advised to be treated, they follow through too.

One in ten women with PID will have fertility issues as a result of scarring in the fallopian tubes, so don't delay being seen out of fear or shame.

CHAPTER 5

Birth Control Basics

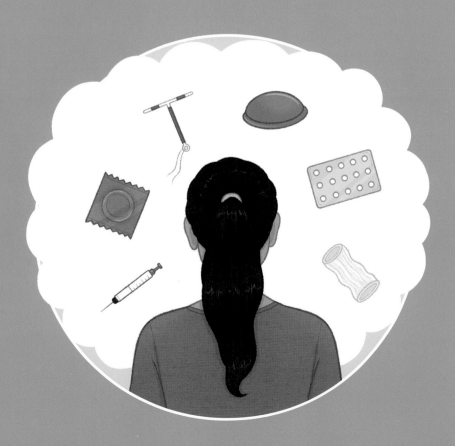

How do I start birth control
without my parents knowing?

In a perfect world, there'd be no need for feeling like you need to keep your birth control usage under wraps. As an OB-GYN, I always advocate for open, honest conversations in families, but I also know that, for some, this conversation just isn't possible.

Parents, this is for you: Thinking that not allowing birth control in your house will keep your teen from having sex is not realistic (as a parent myself, trust me, I'd love to believe this works, just like you). And starting them on birth control won't make them more likely to start having sex—the studies show that's just not true.

So we are left with someone wanting birth control who wants to keep it private. And I respect a patient's right to privacy, especially when they are trying to make sure they do not have a poorly timed pregnancy.

Now, on to accessing birth control.

Depending on your age, state laws can play a role in what you are allowed to access and are able to consent to as a minor. The Guttmacher Institute (guttmacher.org) is a great resource for finding what the laws are state by state.

If you are legally able to access birth control but want to keep it confidential, here are some tips that can help:

- Pay using cash or without insurance (you can look up brands that are less than $5 on your pharmacy of choice's website!).
- Ask for free samples from your doctor or school nurse.
- Look up clinics such as Planned Parenthood or other Title X-funded clinics, which often have free or discounted birth control (including options like IUD and the arm implant!).
- Use online mail-order birth control services (confirm they will not use insurance, or ask how they bill it).
- If you want to use your parents' insurance, call the insurance company to ask how it may be kept confidential on their statements.

Does getting an
IUD insertion hurt?

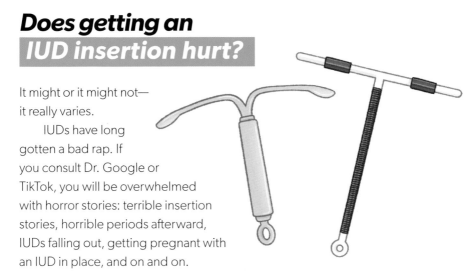

It might or it might not—
it really varies.

IUDs have long
gotten a bad rap. If
you consult Dr. Google or
TikTok, you will be overwhelmed
with horror stories: terrible insertion
stories, horrible periods afterward,
IUDs falling out, getting pregnant with
an IUD in place, and on and on.

Sure, these things can happen, but they are rare. The vast majority
of people who have no issues with their IUDs don't go on the internet to make
boring posts about how uneventful their birth control is. Basically, you're
getting the horror highlights. Like that one friend who has to tell their terrible
birth story to any pregnant person within hearing distance.

So, back to the question: The typical pain associated with having an IUD
placed is cramping, and most folks do great with it. The entire insertion from
start to finish takes on average less than five minutes, so it is very quick.

Cramping can happen at three separate points during the procedure
when your doctor:

- Uses a tool to grasp the outside of your cervix
- Measures the depth of your uterus with a thin device called a uterine
  sound
- Actually places the IUD

And some cramping can continue for about a day afterward.

Lots of studies have been done on the optimal pain control for IUD
placements, with mixed results. I often recommend naproxen (Aleve) a few
hours before insertion, as this medication has some data behind it for helping

with the cramping after the insertion. If you are worried you might need more than this to get through it, don't hesitate to talk with your doctor about a game plan.

Be reassured that many people report having an IUD placed was not as bad as they anticipated! In fact, one study confirmed that a higher level of anxiety, fear of pain, or negative opinions about IUDs was associated with more pain—meaning that a more positive outlook and positive self-talk can actually help you feel *less* pain!

Can I use an IUD
if I haven't had a baby?

You sure can, and if there's one thing that causes my blood pressure to skyrocket, it's when I hear patients telling me that their doctor wouldn't "let" them have an IUD because they haven't given birth before.

That is 100 percent false.

In studies that have looked at IUD placement in women who haven't given birth before versus those who have, there was *no difference* in the success rate of being able to place it.

Rates of the IUD falling out (called expulsion) are exactly the same in people who have birthed versus those who haven't.

And as I discuss on page 117, NO form of birth control causes infertility, so the belief that IUDs make it harder to get pregnant in the future and therefore should be avoided in those with no kids can be taken off the table.

Why, then, does this myth persist?

Honestly, I'm not sure. My guess is it is a lack of ongoing education and is likely spread by older doctors who practiced when we had different IUDs that did at that time cause some problems (today's generation of IUDs are completely different in their safety profile!).

I also think some physicians may think they will be harder to insert, so why not just recommend a different form of birth control? That isn't true, and taking IUDs—an amazingly effective form of birth control that prevents pregnancy over 99 percent of the time—out of the conversation is not fair to patients.

If your doctor says you shouldn't have an IUD because you haven't given birth, you can always gently remind them that the American College of Obstetricians and Gynecologists and the American Academy of Pediatrics disagree—or you can get a second opinion.

Do antibiotics
mess with birth control?

Myth: Antibiotics cancel out your birth control
Fact: Only one kind of antibiotic, rifampin, has been definitively proven to mess up your birth control.

I know, I know—you are going to tell me . . .
- "But my doctor told me I had to use condoms when I was prescribed doxycycline!"
- "Then why does my pharmacist say that's wrong?"
- "We learned differently in nursing school, so . . ."
- "BUT IT SAYS SO ON THE PACKAGE INSERT. WHERE DID YOU GO TO MEDICAL SCHOOL?!"

Here's my answer:
- The studies that suggest antibiotics interfere with birth control were flawed: too small, retrospective, multiple potential biases. This is science speak for "crappy studies make crappy results."
- The most recent study we have shows a *slightly* increased rate of pregnancy with some antibiotics, but it was a rate that went from 6 pregnancies per 100,000 women to 119 per 100,000 women—statistically, this is miniscule. This study also had some flaws.
- Medicolegal fear: "If my patient gets pregnant, she will sue me, so *just in case* I will tell her to use a backup method."
- Maybe the most important: The data we do have on how these drugs are metabolized show NO EFFECT on your birth control whatsoever.

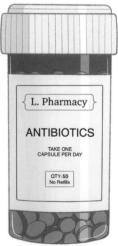

L. Pharmacy

ANTIBIOTICS

TAKE ONE
CAPSULE PER DAY

QTY: 50
No Refills

All of this places birth control pill users in the uncomfortable spot of feeling they are better off safe than sorry, based on flawed information. This extra worry creates a lot of extra burden. Add in alarmist pharmacists and doctors and you've got even more to contend with.

That isn't fair.

We need to demand better labeling, better studies, better counseling (that is not inflammatory or overstates the data), willingness to move on from old myths, and—in the end—shared decision-making.

We deserve better.

Does melatonin "cancel out" my birth control?

Nope. I'm not even going to entertain this one.

I never knew this was a "thing" until I joined TikTok and saw how many posts there were about this. And they all seemed so darn sure that I found myself frantically texting other OB-GYNs I knew and those with whom I had trained. Did I fall asleep that day in residency (haha, sleep, get it?!).

Turns out I hadn't, because it's totally false.

I dove into the research . . . and I came up empty.

So much of what is cited as "evidence" are interviews with doctors on websites that are . . . let's put this kindly, not exactly scientific. I'm talking your everyday pop news websites that are fun to read but should in no way be taken as the voice of hardcore science.

According to the hype, melatonin could hypothetically lead to birth control failure because it is metabolized by the liver, and since birth control is, too, using both could overwhelm the liver, and your BC may not get metabolized properly.

My friends, do you realize how much of a logical leap that is? We don't tell people on birth control to not have a glass of wine (which is metabolized by the liver) or take Tylenol if needed (same deal), so why is melatonin the one thing that is shutting down your BC?

If there should be any counseling about melatonin and birth control, it's that people taking both may actually have higher than average levels of melatonin, so they may need a *lower* dose of the sleep aid than those who are not on birth control.

As long as you wake up when you need to take your pill, you're covered.

Do I have to take my pill the
same time every day?

Nope.

OK, before you start taking it at completely random times, check out the table below.

PROGESTERONE-ONLY NORETHINDRONE PILLS "THE MINI PILL"	PROGESTERONE–ESTROGEN PILLS "THE COMBO PILL"
• Need to be taken in the same 3-hour window • Anything more than 3 hours is considered a missed dose.	• Ideal to take around the same time every day to help with habit, but you've got wiggle room. • At the very least in the same 24-hour period—but aim for a tighter window.

So, while it doesn't need to be exactly the same time every day, trying to shoot for a standard timeframe can be ideal because it gets you into a good habit. You can link it up with brushing your teeth in the morning or use a reminder app to alert you when you're due.

Why do I think this is important to highlight? Because for years people have been scared that they had to take their pill at the exact same nanosecond daily or they'd immediately end up pregnant . . . and that is not based on *any* science. It just adds more stress and guilt—like we need more of *that*—and might make the pills seem more difficult than they are.

Can I just use
condoms?

Absolutely you can!

You just need to understand the statistics and potential pregnancy risks.

Condoms are 87 percent effective at preventing pregnancy with typical use. That number is 98 percent with perfect use, but since no one is truly perfect . . . I think you should be a realist and go with the more realistic number.

Being perfect requires:

- Not storing in wallets or where there is heat (like a glove box)
- Not using oil-based products or lubes (causes tears)
- Using one EVERY time
- Checking the expiration and for tears every time (see page 116 to see how to check)
- Putting them on correctly
- Putting them on before ANY penis–vulva contact
- Taking them off correctly

I think a better way to understand pregnancy risk is to think long term. Here's a table to help you understand that:

PREGNANCIES PER 100 PEOPLE AFTER USING CONDOMS FOR X YEARS:		
	1 year	5 years	10 years
Typical use	21	69	91
Perfect use	5	23	40

So that means if 100 people rely on condoms alone for birth control over 1 year, 21 of them will become pregnant with typical use. Eek!

If those numbers are OK to you, and you accept that risk—then, yes, using condoms alone is fine! But if you want better protection from pregnancy, adding something more effective may be the way to go.

Remember, condoms are still our best tool at preventing STIs in sexually active people, so even though they may not be the best at preventing pregnancy, they still have an important role in the bedroom!

How do I know if a
condom is OK to use?

Use this checklist, and your condom is cleared for takeoff:

[ ]   Check the expiration date.

[ ]   Check packaging for damage (feel for air in package when you squeeze it—if there's none, it's been opened/punctured).

[ ]   Open carefully so it doesn't tear.

[ ]   Put it on before the penis *ever* touches you.

[ ]   Check the direction for unrolling before it touches the penis.

[ ]   Use a new one every time.

And here are some tips to help optimize your condom usage:

- Put some lube inside the condom to help it slide on easier.
- Don't use oil-based lubes (coconut oil, Vaseline, massage oil, hand lotions) with condoms—they cause breakage!
- Flavored condoms can contain sugars that can lead to vaginal yeast infections.
- Do not leave them in wallets or your glove box—damage can result from heat and being handled often.

Will birth control make it harder to
become pregnant when I'm older?

I'll jump right to it: no!

We have absolutely *no studies* that link birth control use of any kind with infertility once you stop using it.

It doesn't matter if you've taken a birth control pill for 15 years or if you had an IUD for a decade—none of these make it harder to get pregnant once you want to.

This is a common myth, so don't feel bad if you've believed this one before.

Here's something many women aren't aware of—taking birth control can actually help *protect* your fertility. Here's how:

1. By thickening cervical mucus, birth control makes it harder for germs like gonorrhea and chlamydia to get into the uterus and cause infection. These infections are linked to infertility, so think of BC as a kind of roadblock.

2. Some forms of birth control are used to treat endometriosis and—you guessed it—by doing so also decrease your risk of endometriosis-associated infertility.

3. BC actually decreases your chances of having an ectopic pregnancy. Having an ectopic pregnancy makes you more likely to have one in the future, so this is another way BC can safeguard your future baby-making plans.

Caveat #1: It can take longer to get your cycle back when you come off the Depo shot. Up to a year is normal.

Caveat #2: If you had abnormal cycles to begin with and that's why you started birth control, then once you stop BC those problems might still be there. That isn't a birth control problem but rather an underlying medical issue. So if this is you, see your doctor and be proactive so you can optimize your fertility when you're ready to make some babies.

Which birth control will make me gain weight?

The *only* birth control method that has been shown to potentially be linked with possible weight gain is the Depo-Provera shot. That's it.

And here are some facts about weight gain on Depo so you can make an informed choice:

- 1 out of 4 women will gain weight on Depo.
- That means 3 out of 4 *don't* gain weight.
- They usually gained 5 percent or more of their body weight in the first 6 months of use.
- Being obese to start with puts you at higher risk for weight gain.
- We think that weight gain is a result of increased appetite, not abnormal metabolism.

So if you're someone who thinks Depo will work best for you and you are worried about weight gain, I want you to know it is not necessarily going to be an issue. It is more likely if you are already overweight, so you may want to reconsider if that's you—but even then, with good food choices and exercise, you can still potentially avoid any changes on the scale.

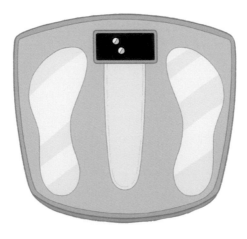

Now, as for all the other birth control methods? There is no proven link to weight gain. I know you might not believe that given what you've heard and what you've seen on social media, but it's true.

On average, adults gain from 0.5 to 1.5 pounds each year. So if you were on the pill for five years, you can see how it'd be easy to say that those extra 5 or so pounds were from BC, right? But it hasn't panned out when we've studied it so far.

Now, if you swear you are seeing crazy weight gain with the start of a birth control method, should you ignore it and not tell your doctor because of what I wrote here? No, of course not!

Absolutely feel free to discuss it, and maybe you still decide to switch up your BC—I fully acknowledge that every person is unique. I will also fully disclose that we could use better studies in this area. Our data is not uber strong, so can an individual user see a difference? It's possible.

What I *don't* want, though, is anyone to avoid a birth control they'd otherwise pick for fear of weight gain because of a misinformed post on social media. Arm yourself with facts!

Because you know what we are 100 percent sure causes lots of weight gain? Pregnancy.

Will birth control
mess with my sex drive?

It is possible that birth control can affect your desire for sex:
- For some users, it may decrease their sex drive.
- For others, it may increase it (taking away a fear of pregnancy can be quite the turn-on).
- And still others—the majority, actually—see no change.

Studies have looked at this and have found that some forms of hormonal birth control can lower sex drive in women using them, but, to be honest, the data has been all over the place.

Just like if you think there may be a link between your birth control and depression (see page 122), I believe that if you feel your BC has crashed your sex drive, you should look into it with your doctor. We should always think holistically and see if anything else has changed that could cause this issue. If not—or even if there may be another factor at play but you still want to change your birth control method—then that's what we will do.

Sex drive isn't an on/off thing—I probably don't need to tell you that. It can be complicated, so if you come off your birth control and are still struggling, don't hesitate to let your doctor know. We can discuss things like individual or couples therapy, sex therapy, or other ideas to help you get the spark back.

Can birth control
help my acne?

Yes, some can.

Combined birth control pills (those with a form of estrogen and progesterone) decrease the amount of androgens that are made by your ovaries. This can be great because androgens are a hormone associated with acne. Lower androgen levels = less acne.

Different combined pills contain different kinds of progesterone, and depending on what form they contain, they may be more effective with keeping acne under control. It's definitely something worth discussing with your OB-GYN or dermatologist when choosing a pill with this goal in mind.

Other forms of birth control that have the same kinds of hormones as the combined pills but are delivered to the body in different forms (such as the patch or vaginal ring) may not be as effective for acne control because of how they are metabolized.

Progesterone-only pills (aka the mini pill) haven't been found to be as effective when compared to the combined type of pill, so you may not want to go this route if clearing up your skin is your goal.

Will birth control
make me depressed?

I can't say for sure, but it is something worth being aware of as a potential possibility.

Many studies that have looked at this have either found no increased risk of depression, or that the data is too difficult to interpret. And it's true—most of the studies we have are too variable to group them all together and draw one big conclusion.

However, a Danish study done in 2016 might be the best information on birth control and depression we have yet, and that is because of its size. It included over 1 million patients! This is because Denmark has a single health care system, which is a *dream* when it comes to data collection.

This study showed a small but noticeable increase in depression in those who use hormonal birth control. A baseline rate of depression was about 1.7 in 100 of those not using birth control compared to 2.2 in 100 of those that did.

In my opinion, that is a *very* tiny increase and not one that should keep a person from using birth control if they want to. However, it can be worth flagging, particularly in people who tend toward depression.

I will also tell you that I don't care what the studies say—if you believe your birth control is messing with your mood, your doctor should know. We can dive into it and see if there might be anything else at play. If not, there is absolutely no harm in switching or stopping hormonal birth control and seeing what happens. Your mental health is important.

Of course, if hormonal BC isn't right for you, finding other ways to prevent pregnancy needs to be discussed because we absolutely know that an unplanned pregnancy can be linked with depression for sure.

What birth control
doesn't have any hormones?

Here are your hormone-free options, with a little info to help you decide if they might be right for you:

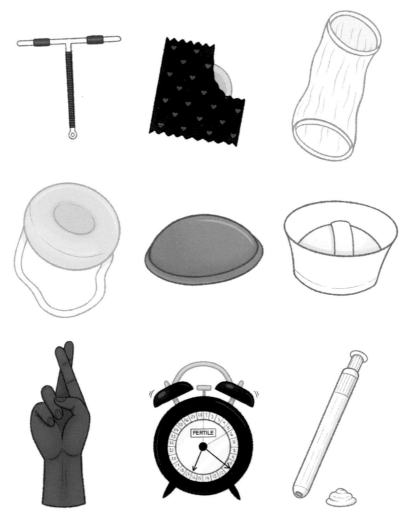

	EFFECTIVENESS AT PREGNANCY PREVENTION (TYPICAL USE)	REQUIRES A DOCTOR'S VISIT?	NOTES
Copper IUD	99.2%	Yes	• In the U.S., it is FDA approved for 10 years but is protective for up to 12 years. • Can make periods heavier or more crampy for some users • Also FDA approved as a method of emergency contraception!
Male condom	87%	No	• See pages 114–116 for more info on usage. • Protects against STIs
Internal condom	79%	No	• Protects against most STIs • Can place up to 2 hours before sex
Fertility-awareness method	77–98%	No	• Also called natural family planning • Different methods exist. • Can involve tracking cycles, basal body temperature, cervical mucus, cervical position • MUST have regular cycles to use this method if cycle tracking is part of your method • Apps can be helpful in helping you track—Natural Cycles is the only FDA-cleared app for birth control. • Requires a lot of dedication
Spermicide	79%	No	• Vaginal gel placed before sex • Many different types are available, and how to use varies—read the instructions! • Changes the vaginal pH and inhibits sperm

	EFFECTIVENESS AT PREGNANCY PREVENTION (TYPICAL USE)	REQUIRES A DOCTOR'S VISIT?	NOTES
Sponge	73–86%	No	• Can be placed up to 24 hours before sex • Must be left in place for 6 hours after sex • Works via a physical barrier and by releasing spermicide
Diaphragm	83%	Yes	• Requires a visit for a fitting, after which you'll get a prescription • Must be used with spermicide • Can be placed a few hours before sex • Must be left in place for 6 hours after sex • Can be left in place up to 24 hours • Requires a new fitting after giving birth or weight change of more than 15 lbs.
Cervical cap	71–86%	No	• More effective if you haven't had a baby • Steeper learning curve than the diaphragm • Must be used with spermicide • Can be placed a few hours before sex • Must be left in place for 6 hours after sex • Can be left in place up to 48 hours • Can be dislodged with rough sex or larger penises
Withdrawal aka "pulling out"	80%	No	• You must rely on your partner to be perfect every time. • Possible to get pregnant off of pre-ejaculate

Should I give my body a break from birth control
every once in a while?

You certainly can if you want to, but there is no medical benefit to doing so. And the risk of pregnancy is there any time you are having unprotected sex!

If you poke around the internet long enough, you will definitely find hormone and wellness "experts" who claim that long-term birth control use is bad for your body and that taking breaks can help keep your health in check.

These same experts claim that suppressing ovulation for so long is frighteningly dangerous for your body. I guess they forgot the part where ovulation suppression (via BC, the pill) actually decreases your risk of ovarian cancer.

They also fail to notice that *in no time in history* have we ever ovulated this much: In ye olden days, we were pregnant constantly from the age of 13 or 14 until we died at the ripe age of 25 (probably during childbirth). Only in modern times have we ever had so many periods, because most of us delay childbearing and live so much longer.

So to summarize: There is no science to support needing birth control "breaks."

We know that long-term birth control usage is safe. There is no link to infertility (see page 117), and it won't affect what your periods are like once you do stop birth control.

In short, this is completely unnecessary.

Enjoy your protection from pregnancy as long as you like!

Do I need a
birth control cleanse?

Why does everything need a cleanse these days? The colon . . . the gut . . . and, apparently, your uterus?!

No, you do not need a birth control cleanse.

Once you stop using whatever form of birth control you were on, consider yourself "cleansed" from it. For almost all methods (other than the Depo-Provera shot), ovulation and fertility jump right back to your baseline. For Depo, it can take up to a year, and that is normal and expected.

Since I was never trained in cleanses of the birth control kind, I turned to my trusty online hormone experts who promote these and—wouldn't you just know it?!—they sell the very products that will "cleanse" you.

They've even given this "pre-cleanse" state a name: post–birth control syndrome. Now *that* is some savvy doctoring, inventing conditions that you alone have the expertise, and products, to treat.

These, ahem, experts state that after coming off birth control you can "reset" your body with their programs and supplements to help your mood, skin, and libido. Brain fog? Hair loss? Crazy periods? According to them, it's all because you came off BC, so you'd better get on your cleanse.

These programs cost hundreds of dollars. And there is no science to support them. It is maddening.

I want you to skip the cleanses and the detoxes and spend that money on more fun things, or at the very least, evidence-based things.

And I want you to see your doctor if you notice any issues when you come off your BC. Remember—as we age, our cycles can change, and if you were on the pill for 10 years, sure, they could be different when you stop. If you went on BC because your period was miserable, you may experience that when you stop too. Check in with your doctor if you have concerns before you turn to these internet "experts."

Regardless, you don't need a cleanse. Please don't give your money to these charlatans who profit off people in this way.

Are online companies that
ship birth control legit?

They sure are, and they can be a great way to get your BC without ever having to leave home!

There are a multitude of online birth control companies that are legitimate and can be trusted. Some offer just the pill, while others also carry the patch, vaginal ring, emergency contraception, and even treatment for herpes outbreaks. Fantastic!

In general, these companies have women's health care providers on staff who can review your history and make sure you are a good candidate for birth control before it is prescribed. They might do this via an electronic form or a phone call. Insurance coverage is often available, so you can check and see if they take yours (and if not, they often have affordable generics).

Depending on medical and dispensing licenses, these companies may not be able to ship birth control to every state—so that is another important thing to check when scoping out which company may be the best fit for you.

If you are worried about other people in your household finding out that you are on birth control, you can rest assured that discretion is key with these companies. Most will ship your BC in a package that doesn't give away what is hidden inside. If you are using family insurance, however, you do want to reach out to the company to ask how your prescription may show up on insurance billing. They can walk you through different options.

If you think it seems weird that birth control can be prescribed this way, it may be helpful to know that the American College of Obstetricians and Gynecologists supports birth control being made over the counter. Studies have shown that those with a uterus can use self-screening tools to determine if they are cleared for BC use without any compromise to safety, and we OB-GYNs would love to see improved access in this way. Needing to go see a doctor for a birth control prescription is a huge barrier to access.

For now, some states allow pharmacists to prescribe it directly. Between that and online birth control companies, the hope is that everyone will have better access to birth control while we continue to advocate for OTC status. Happy online shopping!

Is it OK to not have a period
while on birth control?

Absolutely. In fact, that is the main reason some people go on birth control in the first place—they hate having periods.

It can be confusing to hear this when we say the opposite is true if you are *not* on birth control. That is, not having periods—or having very irregular, infrequent ones—when not on birth control can be cause for concern and should be investigated. It could be associated with hormonal issues like thyroid disorders, PCOS, or other problems that, if left untreated, can put you at higher risk for infertility or cancer of the uterus.

While on birth control, however, not having a period is perfectly fine. This is because many forms of birth control work by keeping the lining of the uterus so thin that there is nothing to bleed or shed every month. Also, by suppressing ovulation, your body doesn't have the usual cycle of hormonal ups and downs that can trigger a period.

Not having a period while on birth control is *not* a sign that you will struggle with infertility when you come off your BC. This is an important note, since many of us have been told the opposite is true.

All in all, not having a period can be a very enjoyable side effect of birth control for many users. If you are someone who likes having your period (for some uterus owners it can be very reassuring, as it lets them know they aren't pregnant, for example), be sure to discuss that desire with your doctor before selecting your form of birth control.

Does alcohol or CBD affect birth control?

Alcohol does not change how well your birth control works, unless you are so drunk you forget to take your pill or use a condom . . . or you throw up your pill.

If you take your pill and throw up within two hours, you should consider that a missed pill and take another one ASAP. If you were on your placebo week, don't worry about replacing those—they have no hormones in them so there is no need to take a replacement.

If you forgot to use a condom or otherwise had unprotected sex (say you forgot to put in your diaphragm or your partner was drunk and didn't pull out in time), then you should consider emergency contraception if you want to prevent pregnancy. See page 163 for information about your EC options and which one might be best for you. You should also consider STI testing if a condom wasn't used.

As for CBD, the science on how this drug interacts with many medications is still in its infancy. Studies have shown that CBD is metabolized by an enzyme class called cytochrome P450, the same group of enzymes that breaks down birth control pills. Some studies have suggested CBD may decrease the efficacy of birth control, while others say it may actually prevent birth control breakdown and therefore increase its dose in the blood stream, possibly increasing some side effects risks.

The bottom line on CBD? We don't know enough yet. Talk to your doctor if you take the pill and decide what is right for you, personally, considering your health, risks, benefits, and alternatives.

Why isn't there a
`birth control pill for men?!`

I hear you loud and clear on this one. Wouldn't it be nice if just for once men had to take the reins on birth control?

Right now, the only options for cis men to prevent pregnancy are condoms or a vasectomy. That is sadly it (I'm not even going to count withdrawal because that is so unreliable).

So why don't we have better BC for men? Unfortunately, there's a problem—actually, millions of them. Here's a staggering fact: Men can produce about 1,500 sperm per second. EACH SECOND of every day, 24/7. That's impressive.

Suppressing ovulation is one of the mainstays of birth control—and with some hormonal changes delivered via a medication, it isn't that hard to prevent a once-a-month event. But shutting down an entire system of sperm production that happens on a daily basis? That is a lot more difficult.

Since men aren't the ones actually getting pregnant, regulating agencies are much stricter when it comes to side effects they may experience from the birth control. Since they aren't the ones who would actually get pregnant and give birth (and experience the side effects and risks from those events), any side effects they might get from birth control are scrutinized much more closely—meaning it might be harder to get a medication approved for them.

Here are some current options under investigation:

- A one-time gel that is injected into the vas deferens (aka the sperm superhighway) to block the path for sperm. This can then be flushed out when trying to conceive.
- A topical gel that contains a hormone like progestin and testosterone that is rubbed daily onto the skin to decrease sperm production.
- A daily pill containing progestin and testosterone to decrease sperm production.

These options still have a long way to go before becoming mainstream, unfortunately. So far, these hormonal methods take three to four months to become effective, so they still require quite a bit of waiting.

Studies are promising, but we have a long way to go.

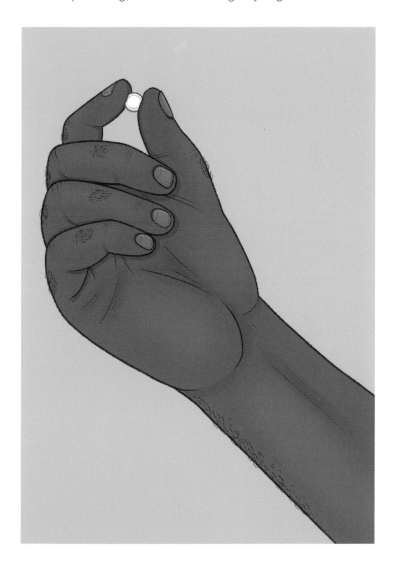

CHAPTER 6
Going to the Doctor

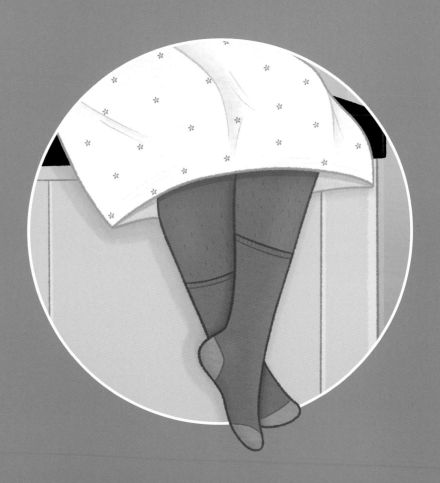

Will my doctor do a
pelvic exam at my first visit?

Not necessarily.

It's OK to feel nervous about a pelvic exam—and we will dive into that more on page 148—but it can help to know they aren't an automatic every time you see an OB-GYN.

Unless you have the concerns I listed on page 144, at your first visit, it is likely you won't need a pelvic exam at all.

Lots of people think you have to have a pelvic exam to be prescribed birth control. Let me say this loud and clear: Pelvic exams are NOT needed to start you on birth control unless you are using certain kinds when it's physically necessary (like an IUD or diaphragm). Seriously.

The American College of Obstetricians and Gynecologists supports this— so your birth control should *not* be held hostage by a pelvic exam if you are healthy and don't have a medical reason to need one.

If your doctor wants to do a pelvic exam, but you are not feeling it, it is OK to say no. You and your doctor can discuss the risks versus the benefits. Truly, it may be in your best interest to have one—but at the end of the day, you should never feel forced. I've got some tips on page 148 on how to make exams easier if you need a confidence boost.

Do pelvic exams
hurt?

They should not, and if they do, you should let your doctor know so they can stop.

Pressure and slight cramping can be expected. Pain is a reason to speak up and ask for a time-out.

If you are having pain, your doctor can try:

- Using a smaller speculum
- Going more slowly
- Adjusting the angle of the speculum
- Talking you through the exam
- Encouraging you to take deep breaths and relax your muscles more

Still in pain? It might be time to stop for the day.

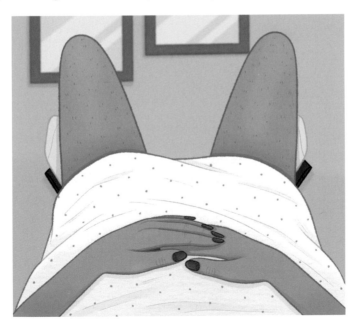

Some people who experience a lot of pain with pelvic exams may have conditions such as:

- Pelvic floor myalgia or vaginismus (think tense pelvic muscles that aren't under conscious control)
- Vulvar pain disorders
- Endometriosis
- History of trauma
- Anxiety

For these folks, taking a deep breath may not cut it. If this is you, you can talk with your doctor about some techniques that might help—I cover a bunch on page 148.

Can I go to the
OB-GYN without telling my parents?

Yes, you can see a doctor by yourself, but let's cover what that includes.

In the United States, every state is different and has its own set of laws for minors (those under 18 years old) to consent to different things. This is super annoying—because how you get to care for your body should *not* depend on where you live. But here we are.

As with the laws on accessing birth control for minors mentioned on page 106, a great resource for various state laws is the Guttmacher Institute (guttmacher.org), specifically these pages:

- "Minors' access to contraceptive services"
- "An overview of consent to reproductive health services by young people"

You can also check your local Planned Parenthood website.

Here are a few important highlights:

- Minors can request STI testing in all 50 states (yay!) . . .
- . . . but in 18 states, their doctor can inform the patient's parents if they think it is in the teen's best interest (boo!).
- Only 23 states allow *all* minors to consent to birth control, while others require certain conditions. (See the Guttmacher Institute website for much more on this.)

Then there is the issue of billing. Your visit can show up on your parents' insurance if you use that to pay for it. If you don't want that to happen, you can:

- Pay with cash.
- Go to a free clinic.
- Ask your doctor how things can be written in your chart so that the nature of your visit won't be clear in an insurance statement.
- Call your insurance and ask if they are able to keep things confidential.

You also need to ask your doctor if your parents have access to your records. This is most important if your doctor uses electronic records and your parents can access them from home.

Bottom line: Research what you state allows, and then talk to your doctor about your confidentiality concerns.

I am always a fan of being honest and open with parents, but I'm also realistic that that isn't always possible. I cover more about this in the next section, so keep reading.

Can my doctor
tell my parents what we talked about?

As doctors, we are bound by confidentiality (meaning we keep your stuff private) within the scope of the law. We *are* obligated to tell others if you share with us that you want to harm yourself or someone else. This isn't to make life hard for you but instead to get you the care you need (if you are suicidal) or prevent harm to others.

When it comes to whether you are sexually active or want to start birth control or screen for STIs, rules about reporting your private information all depend on where you live. See the websites on page 139 to check your state's laws.

Remember: In some states, your doctor *can* tell your parents what has happened during your visit if they think it is in your best interest. I want to ask that you *not* let that be a reason you keep important information from us. Be honest and tell us you that you don't want us to tell your parents—we may determine that it is actually *better* for your health (mental and physical) if we keep it between us.

We can work together as a team to decide how we help you best.

Will my doctor be able to
tell if I've had sex?

We can only know if you've had sex if you tell us . . . or if you're pregnant.

There is no virginity test and no way for us to tell from an examination.

Many people think the appearance of the hymen is a dead giveaway about someone's virginity status, but the truth is, hymens vary. Some are noticeable. Others aren't. Some tear from non-sexual activities like riding a bike or being active.

I repeat: You cannot rely on the appearance of the hymen or a pelvic examination to know if someone is sexually active.

The World Health Organization even issued a statement saying that "virginity testing" is completely inaccurate and is a "violation of the victim's human rights." I couldn't agree more.

Do I have to get a
pap smear?

Lots of folks hear about getting a pap smear when they talk about their sexual health. A pap smear is part of a pelvic exam, and it's important to understand what each one is (and isn't).

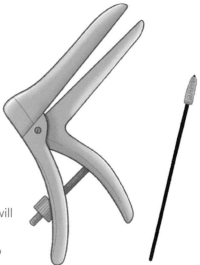

Pelvic exam: an exam where your doctor will do four things:

1. Look at the outside of your vulva to make sure the skin is healthy.
2. Place a speculum into the vagina to look at the vagina and cervix.
3. Potentially collect some specimens for testing (for infections or for a pap smear).
4. Remove the speculum and insert two fingers vaginally while placing a hand on your belly to make sure the uterus and ovaries feel normal.

SPECULUM

an instrument (pictured above) that is placed inside the vagina that allows your doctor to see the vagina and cervix. They can be made out of plastic or metal.

PAP SMEAR

Done as part of a pelvic exam, its purpose is to collect cells from your cervix so they can be looked at under the microscope to scan for precancerous or cancerous cells. We often do a cervical swab for certain strains of HPV (human papillomavirus) at the same time, since these can lead to cervical cancer.

So, if your question is do you need a pelvic exam when you see your OB-GYN, the answer is *maybe*. Reasons we do pelvic exams include:

- Pap smear or STI testing (some STI tests are done this way, but not all)
- Abnormal vaginal discharge
- Abnormal vaginal bleeding
- Abdominal or pelvic pain
- IUD insertion
- Monitoring for growths like fibroids or cysts

And if it's the pap smear you are asking about, the answer is *maybe* (again). See the next page, where I discuss how often you need screening.

Don't worry: You aren't alone if you've always thought pap smears and pelvic exams were the same thing. It is a common misconception!

How long can I go
between pap smears?

Even as I write this, the guidelines may be changing, so I always recommend you discuss this with your doctor.

Current recommendations from the American College of Obstetricians and Gynecologists and the U.S. Services Preventive Task Force recommend:

- **Younger than 21:** No paps
- **21–29 years old:** Every 3 years
- **30–65 years old:** Every 3 years, or every 5 years with an HPV test, or an HPV test every 5 years alone
- **66 or older:** Discuss with your doctor, as you may be able to stop

You might think not getting a pap test every year seems strange, but the evidence shows that it is safe to space them out more when you are negative for the high-risk strains of HPV that are associated with cervical cancers and thus, abnormal pap smears.

Keep in mind that people who have had abnormal paps or have other high-risk conditions may need more frequent screening or screening at an earlier age.

You should still see your OB-GYN every year, however! We do *so* much more than just a pap at your annual exam: blood pressure screening, birth control counseling, breast exams, monitoring for depression, domestic violence, STIs, healthy habits, family planning goals . . . the list goes on!

Do lesbians need
pap smears?

Yes.

Some people—including some health care professionals—erroneously think that women who have sex with women do not need pap smears. They assume that this population has not been exposed to HPV from men and thus are not at risk for cervical cancer.

These assumptions are wrong, and they have led to queer women receiving far fewer cervical cancer screenings than their heterosexual counterparts.

An assigned female at birth who only has sex with other assigned females at birth may have had sex with a man at some point, and therefore she could have been exposed to HPV that way. We also know that while it may be less likely, HPV can spread from woman to woman during sex, either directly or with the use of toys.

Pap tests should be done on the same schedule for all people with a cervix—see page 145—regardless of their sexual orientation.

What do I do if my
doctor doesn't listen to me?

If you feel you are not being heard, it is probably time to move on to a new doctor.

A doctor–patient relationship is supposed to be a partnership. Both people are supposed to work together to keep you healthy. When it comes to your parts down there, I think it's even more important you feel like your doctor is on your side and has your back.

Feeling like things are a bit offtrack, but you want to stick it out? It's important to speak up. You might say:

- "I'm not sure you are hearing what is worrying me."
- "I feel like I am not getting across my concerns."
- "I would like to discuss some alternative ideas about ___."

Still not making the connection? It's OK to move on to another provider.

If you feel that your provider was inappropriate and would like to report that, you can always ask to speak with a practice manager or patient advocate. More concerning issues can be brought in front of state or hospital medical boards.

Your voice and your health matter.

What if I feel triggered by the
thought of going to the OB-GYN?

Many people who have experienced trauma in the past feel triggered at the thought of reexperiencing anything that resembles their previous trauma. For survivors of sexual trauma, merely speaking of sex and body parts, and certainly an exam of private parts, can trigger horrible memories.

I am so sorry you experienced something that causes such a response. My purpose in this section is to provide tools to help anyone who finds going to the OB-GYN difficult feel equipped to take their power back.

Some or all of these suggestions may help make it easier for you:

- **Let your doctor know.** If we know, we can discuss how to make you more comfortable.
- **Let's just talk first.** No need for an exam on that first visit—it's OK to spend that time getting to know each other and making a plan for when you do need an exam.
- **Bring a friend.** A support person who can be there during the exam can be your advocate and stand by your side when you need it most. A nurse or medical assistant at the practice can also be that person for you.
- **Maybe a distraction?** For some, having headphones to listen to music or watching a YouTube video gets them through it. For others, the need to be totally aware is important.
- **What do you want from us?** Do you want me to tell you everything I'm going to do before I do it or be quiet and not bother you? Does having an unrelated conversation help (I will talk about WHATEVER you want!)?
- **Do you need to take medication**? For some survivors, taking an antianxiety medication is necessary, and that is OK. Just make sure any paperwork that needs signing is done beforehand and that you have a ride home.
- **Stop means stop**. Let your doctor know that when you say stop, they stop. No questions asked.

Learning to be able to get through pelvic exams after trauma can actually be very empowering. We will work together to find what works for you—because you are worth it.

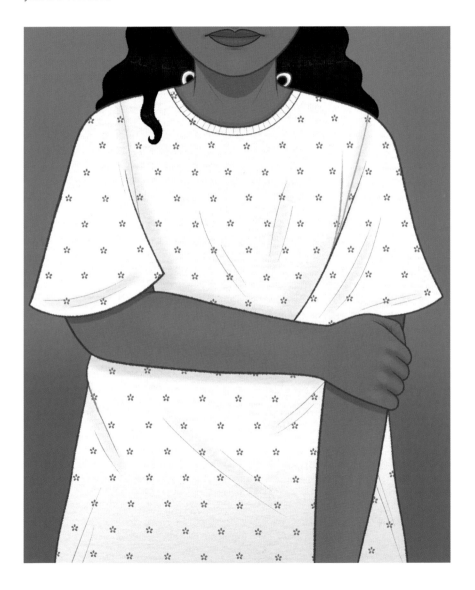

Can I ask my doctor to
check for a hormone imbalance?

You can, but more than likely we will recommend against it.

Let's consider a scenario I've seen play out for some patients:

Jane establishes care with a provider who advertises a holistic approach and treating ailments with natural remedies. During her visit, Jane discusses how she has felt more tired and bloated lately, and sex with her boyfriend of three years is no longer as exciting. Her naturopath recommends checking her hormones to make sure they are "balanced" and recommends an online test that costs $399. This blood and saliva test measures her levels of estrogen, progesterone, testosterone, thyroid studies, and a few other hormones. Jane's naturopath calls and tells her that her results show estrogen dominance and believes it is the cause of her symptoms. She is told to change to a vegetarian diet and start on probiotics and other supplements that the naturopath can sell her for $200 a month. She also recommends she stop using her birth control pills, stating that it is worsening her symptoms and causing inflammation in her body.

So, hormone imbalances: Are they something we can diagnose with some tests and then treat?

Most mainstream doctors will say no. Testing hormones with saliva is not at all accurate—levels can vary greatly by time of day and depending on what you've eaten. Saliva tests are not considered a reliable measure of the actual hormone levels in your body. Even blood testing for hormones is not much better, since we see normal daily fluctuations.

The vast majority of those who promote testing for hormone imbalances are people who then want to or are connected to someone who sells you something to "fix" this imbalance—and that is a huge ethical red flag. For example, one popular online practitioner claims that with her detox program (costing almost $200), you can fix your estrogen dominance in 21 days. Don't forget her women's health balancing supplement (costing $720 for a year's supply), which contains 16,000 percent more vitamin B-12 than the recommended daily dietary intake. Yikes.

If it sounds too good to be true, it probably is.

If you have symptoms that are bothering you and you think it's related to hormones, let's talk about it. Your doctor should take a thoughtful history, do an exam, and may order some testing—but, despite what you'll find advertised online, hardly ever is it caused by imbalanced hormones.

Can my doctor
test me for endometriosis?

ENDOMETRIOSIS

a condition when the endometrium (or uterine lining cells) are found outside the uterus, such as on the ovaries, fallopian tubes, or elsewhere in the abdomen and pelvis.

Unfortunately, there is no definitive test for endometriosis other than surgery, but we don't always want to jump to this straight away. That doesn't mean we can't make an educated attempt at a diagnosis without it, however.

If you have painful periods, pain with sex, abdominal or pelvic pain, then endometriosis can be on the short list of suspects. Other symptoms such as back pain with your period, diarrhea, constipation, pain with bowel movements or urinating can be suspicious too, though they are a bit less specific.

If your doctor suspects endometriosis, an attempt to suppress the endometriosis lesions by using medications such as birth control or other hormonal treatments can not only help your symptoms but also help clarify the diagnosis.

If this doesn't work, or if you would like to try to get pregnant, then your doctor may recommend surgery. This is usually a laparoscopic (minimally invasive) surgery where your doctor will look in your abdomen and pelvis for any suspicious lesions. If seen, they can be ablated, or better yet, removed and sent to the lab where a pathologist can look under a microscope and confirm if they were truly caused by endometriosis or not.

Endometriosis is common, affecting about 1 in 10 people with a uterus, so don't hesitate to bring up your concerns with your doctor if you think you have the symptoms.

I'm trans/nonbinary/gender diverse—
do I still need to go to a gynecologist?

If you were born with and you still have a uterus, ovaries, a cervix, or breasts/chest tissue, then you need to see *someone* to keep an eye on those organs, but it doesn't have to be a gynecologist.

For some trans or nonbinary people, the idea of walking into a women's health center is the last thing they want to do. And that is totally OK, because there are lots of people in the medical community who provide care for these organs.

Other providers who can continue these important screenings include family medicine and internal medicine nurse practitioners and physicians, who tend to have spaces that might feel more comfortable.

Before assuming your primary care provider offers cervical cancer screening, however, call and confirm so you aren't disappointed at your visit if they tell you they can't do that. If the idea of having a pelvic exam for cervical cancer screening causes you distress, talk to your provider. They may be able to give you medicine to help calm your anxiety during the exam.

In addition to screening for cervical cancer, you need screening for cancers that can affect other organs as well as STIs. Pregnancy prevention (if desired) as well as monitoring of menstrual cycles is important too.

Many transgender/nonbinary/gender-diverse individuals born with a uterus and ovaries desire biological children or children related to them.

Even individuals who have been on testosterone can stop testosterone and carry a pregnancy or use a gestational carrier for a fetus conceived with their gametes/eggs, and OB-GYNs can assist with these procedures. On the other hand, individuals who are taking testosterone can become pregnant even if they are not having regular cycles, so it is critical to use birth control if you have intercourse with individuals who produce sperm.

If gender-affirming surgery is something you are interested in, there are many OB-GYNs and plastic and reconstructive surgeons who offer these services and are well versed in providing respectful, inclusive care. At that time, you can also make a plan for how to continue your regular health screens moving forward.

Do I call my doctor if I've
lost a tampon/condom in my vagina?

Don't worry, we can find them!

And you are not alone—I promise it happens more than you think.

For getting these out, try these tips:

- Try to relax!
- Get comfortable either squatting or lying down with your knees bent and out to the side. Sometimes one leg up on the toilet helps too.
- Take a few deep breaths, and with a clean finger reach into the vagina and try to hook out the condom or the tampon string, then grasp and remove.
- Not working? Switch up positions and try again.
- Enlist the help of your partner—sometimes they can get at an angle that you can't.

You can also try to bear down or have a bowel movement and see if that helps—sometimes that downward pressure helps to expel the condom or bring it or the tampon lower to where you can try again to snag it.

Still not happening? Give your doctor or trusty urgent care a call, and we will be happy to help. I promise you are not the first person who's dealt with this! We'll use a speculum to see where it's hiding and use a grasper to get it out.

Important note: If you've got a condom in the vagina, you could be at risk for pregnancy (if it's the only birth control you are using) or sexually transmitted infections. If you don't want to be pregnant, getting a prescription for emergency contraception or buying some over the counter ASAP is important (see page 163 for more on this). You should also be tested for STIs and can talk to your doctor about when to do that.

The one thing you should not do is ignore it. Your risk of infection increases the longer any foreign body is left in place. Don't worry; this is not something to be embarrassed about!

CHAPTER 7

Possibly Pregnant

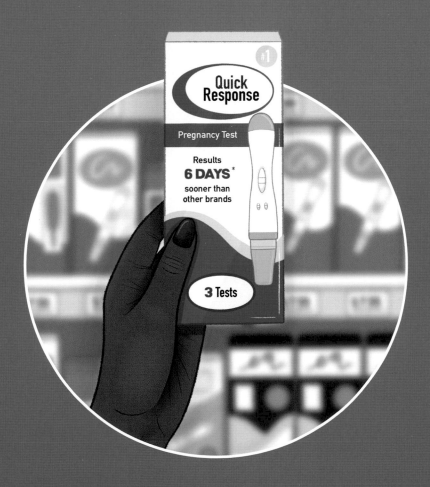

If my partner pulled out, can I still get pregnant?

This is technically called the withdrawal method (aka pulling out), and we in the medical field have another name for this too: impending parenthood.

OK, yes, pulling out is better than when your partner ejaculates inside you in terms of pregnancy prevention. But it's a terrible form of birth control if you *truly* don't want to get pregnant (if you don't mind an "oops" pregnancy, then this method might work for you).

When using this method for birth control, the failure rate is around 20 percent.

That means if 100 of your friends rely on pulling out, approximately 20 will end up pregnant by the end of a year. That's a very high failure rate when it comes to birth control!

Using this method requires that your partner be able to predict exactly when they are about to ejaculate and pull out every time, on time. That can be hard to do in the moment and even more so if you're intoxicated or if your partner isn't as dedicated to maintaining your not-pregnant status as you are.

And remember—with this method, you are putting all your trust into someone *else* being perfect for it to work. Is that control you want to hand over?

The next question is inevitably about pre-cum. That's the fluid that leaks out of the penis prior to ejaculation. We don't have very many studies, but some have shown that there can be some sperm in this fluid—another reason why the withdrawal method isn't that effective.

If you rely on this method, it's not a bad idea to have some emergency contraception in your medicine cabinet in case there is a slip-up.

If there is semen on my partner's hand when he fingers me, can I get pregnant?

Yes. If you've used the withdrawal method or have done some mutual masturbation (when you help each other out or masturbate side-by-side) and your partner has some ejaculate on their fingers, keep them away from your vulva and vagina!

It is definitely possible to get pregnant this way.

It doesn't matter how the sperm gets in your vagina, whether by penis, finger, or turkey baster—once it's there, it has the ability to swim its way through the cervix, into the uterus, and up to your fallopian tubes where it may meet an egg waiting to be fertilized.

Most likely, the risk of pregnancy in this scenario is lower than when ejaculation happens directly into the vagina because there's probably less ejaculate involved. But we don't know how much less, and the average ejaculate has millions of sperm in it—is that a risk you are willing to take?

If you don't want to get pregnant, have your partner stay away from your vulva and out of your vagina if there is semen involved. Or have them wash their hands thoroughly before they say hello. Hand hygiene is never a bad thing!

I think I might be pregnant—
what do I do?

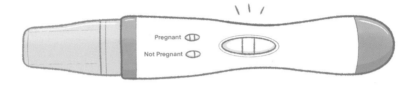

First, take a deep breath.

If you find yourself pregnant and this wasn't a planned situation, your emotions might be all over the map.

Every person who is pregnant has three choices:
1. Continuing the pregnancy and parenting
2. Continuing the pregnancy and adoption
3. Not continuing the pregnancy

It is OK if you don't know what you want to do when you first see those pink lines.

The best thing you can do is give yourself space to think. You may want to talk to your partner (if there is one) or a trusted friend or family member. Seeing your OB-GYN who knows you to discuss next steps can be helpful too.

If you don't have an OB-GYN, or you aren't sure what you want to do, you can certainly seek care at a place like Planned Parenthood or other reproductive health clinics. Contrary to what some people want you to believe, places like Planned Parenthood will discuss all options with you and will *not* push you into making a decision to end your pregnancy. They are in the business of supporting informed choice—not coercion.

In the meantime, if you are considering continuing the pregnancy, taking a prenatal vitamin while you sort things out is a good idea.

If you know you want to be pregnant, go ahead and call your OB-GYN and see when they recommend making your first appointment, and start buying the books and getting excited!

If adoption is something you would consider, your OB-GYN can certainly help give you the names of some local resources for more information. Remember, seeking information and talking to someone about considering adoption doesn't mean you are committing to it.

If you do not want to remain pregnant, it's important to know that laws vary by state in terms of access to services like abortion. You can check out Guttmacher.org or your local Planned Parenthood's website to see what the laws are where you live. Some are very restrictive when it comes to the gestational age of the pregnancy (how far along you are) and when you can have an abortion, so it's important to find that out.

If you find your doctor isn't supportive of your choices—regardless of what they may be—save yourself the headache and find a new one.

Oops! I forgot to use protection and had sex—
what now?

First, breathe. Try not to panic! We've got options, but time is of the essence when it comes to an oopsies with unprotected sex.

Emergency contraception (aka EC) is what is used when the condom breaks or you had sex after missing a few pills, or other related birth control blunders. There are a few different kinds of EC, so read below and see which one might be right for you. It's not just a pill!

EMERGENCY CONTRACEPTION

a type of birth control that is used *after* sex to prevent pregnancy, working by preventing or delaying ovulation. EC does *not* cause an abortion.

Keep in mind the following:
- All methods are more effective the sooner you take them!
- Weight can affect certain types of EC:
  —If you weigh more than 155 pounds, ella is a better choice than the levonorgestrel pill.
  —If you weigh more than 195 pounds, ella may not be as effective— consider the copper IUD.

Want to be the most prepared version of you? Keep Plan B or ella in your medicine cabinet in case you might need it; that way, you'll never be left scrambling!

	COPPER IUD	ULIPRISTAL ACETATE	LEVONORGESTREL	BIRTH CONTROL PILLS
Brand name/ method	Paragard	ella	Plan B Next Choice My Way After Pill . . . and more	Yuzpe method (see below)
Formulation	Intrauterine device	1 tablet	One 1.5 mg tablet or two 0.75 mg tablets	Combination of pills (different protocols for different pills exist)
Effectiveness	99.9%	85%–98%	88–95%	75%
Time frame for use after sex	5 days	5 days	3 days	5 days
Over the counter	No	No	Yes	No
Requires an office visit	Yes	No	No	No

How do I get the morning-after pill or other types of
emergency contraception?

As we just covered in the prior section, there are a few different options when it comes to emergency contraception (EC). When it comes to getting your hands on a version of the morning-after pill, it depends on which kind you are looking to use.

LEVONORGESTREL PILL

The levonorgestrel EC pill, which has many names but is most recognizable by the brand names Plan B (two pills) or Plan B One-Step (one pill), is over the counter. Here are a few tips on how to get it:

- Go to your nearest pharmacy or look online for pharmacies that stock these so you aren't searching when you get to the store. By law, they should be right on the shelves, usually by the condoms and such, but sometimes you may need to ask the pharmacist to get it for you from behind the counter (which is annoying because it is just another barrier).

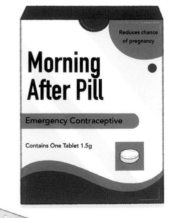

- If a pharmacist refuses to sell these pills to you, demand to speak to their manager and file a report.

- Order online directly from the manufacturer website or trusted online birth control mail-order companies. Personally, I'd stay away from Amazon, as prices that are very cheap may be too good to be true and reports of opened packages have me concerned.

- There is no age limit to who can buy Plan B. Thankfully, this restriction was removed years ago.
- You also don't have to be the person taking it to purchase the EC—so if your partner offers to get it, feel free to take them up on it.

ELLA EC

This does require a prescription, and even though you have a longer window in which to use it, sooner is always better. You can get ella by:

- Calling your doctor and asking for a prescription (calling on weekends and after hours is OK for something like this!)
- Ordering online from a mail-order birth control company (same advice when it comes to sticking with reputable companies). Many will overnight ship them to you.
- Your best bet: have a prescription filled, and keep the pill on hand in case you ever need it! Even having your doctor write a prescription for you to fill when you need it urgently is an option.

Does taking emergency contraception more than once
mess up my body?

While it may lead to some spotting or make the timing of your next period unpredictable, taking emergency contraception (EC) pills will *not* do any lasting harm that we know of, whether you take them once or ten times.

In other words, there is no limit to how many times you can take Plan B or ella. It will not cause infertility, mess up your uterus, give you cancer, or any of the other things I have heard out there. Using it frequently does lead to a higher dose of hormones and probably more irregular cycles, which isn't ideal, but there is no hard data to support a limit on the number of uses.

That said, one of the brand names of EC is called Plan B for a reason! Ideally, you've got something else that is protecting you from pregnancy on a consistent basis rather than relying on emergency contraception all the time. In the long term, emergency contraception is less effective than using regular birth control to prevent pregnancy.

But if you can't do birth control or don't have access to a form of it that works for you, then EC when you need it is better than nothing!

Do I need a pregnancy test *from the doctor?*

Nope—not usually.

The urine pregnancy tests we have in the office and the hospital are not any better than the ones you can buy in the grocery store. In fact, the ones at the dollar store are just as good, so save your money!

If you need a blood pregnancy test—which is only needed if we have concerns for high-risk factors like miscarriage or ectopic pregnancy—then, yes, you'll need to see your doctor for that.

I'm pregnant—and I don't know who the father is.
When can I find out?

This one can be tough. Rest assured you are not alone if this is where you find yourself. There are tests that can be done to determine paternity (who the father is).

Before you decide to do this testing, consider what you will do with this information. For example, would it change your mind about parenting, adoption, or abortion if you did these tests during pregnancy? If not, consider waiting until the baby is born as those tests can be lower risk than more invasive prenatal (during pregnancy) options.

If you do decide to test prenatally, make sure the lab running your tests is accredited by the American Association of Blood Banks, as they are required to adhere to high standards for testing, chain of custody, and reporting. Don't just pick the cheapest option on the internet.

There are two ways to determine who the father is when you are still pregnant. See the following page for the differences of each:

TYPE OF TESTS	INVASIVE TESTING	NONINVASIVE TESTING
AKA	Chorionic villus sampling (CVS) or amniocentesis	Noninvasive prenatal testing (NIPT) or cell-free DNA (cfDNA) testing
How it's done	**CVS:** a small needle is placed through the vagina or abdomen into the placenta to remove a small sample of cells **Amniocentesis:** a needle is passed through the belly into the uterus, and a small amount of amniotic fluid is removed (with fetal cells in it)	A blood sample from the pregnant person is taken (their blood contains some fetal DNA). The potential father has a cheek swab, and both sets of DNA are compared, giving you a percentage of likelihood that they are the dad (0–100%).
Timing in pregnancy	**CVS:** 10–13 weeks of pregnancy **Amniocentesis:** after 15 weeks of pregnancy	10 weeks of pregnancy or later
Risks	• 1–2% risk of bag of water breaking • 1 in 300–1,000 risk of miscarriage	Inability to give results (some cfDNA tests are unable to be interpreted)
Benefits	Sample can also be used to run other screening tests and is considered more accurate for these than noninvasive prenatal testing (NIPT).	• No need for an invasive procedure • The cfDNA can be used for other screening tests
Costs (estimate)	$1,500–2,000	$300–500
Covered by insurance	May not be for determining paternity (genetic screening may be covered)	May not be for determining paternity (genetic screening may be covered)

How do I know if I am
fertile or not?

When it comes to being able to declare you fertile or not, there is no perfect test (though plenty of companies want you to think there is, and they will gladly sell you a kit!). However, we can look for some clues that indicate your fertility.

To get pregnant, you need to ovulate, or release an egg. Signs that you are likely regularly ovulating include:

- Regular cycles (starting your period every 21 to 35 days)
- Ovulation predictor kits giving you positive results
- Cervical mucus that indicates ovulation (see page 30)
- Basal body temperature tracking that shows ovulation
- Blood tests for hormones (like follicle-stimulating hormone, aka FSH, and estrogen) that show ovulation
- An ultrasound showing ovaries that are preparing to ovulate

Ovulation is only one part of the picture, though. How many eggs you have affects your fertility, and this number was set way back when you were in the womb. A blood test for anti-Mullerian hormone (AMH) is nicknamed the ovarian reserve test, because it can give us an idea of how healthy your ovaries are and your number of eggs. This test can only give an estimate, though, and should not be used alone!

None of these tests can predict the health of your uterus or fallopian tubes, or the sperm count and quality of your eventual partner. Worried about your fertility? Chat with your doctor so they can review what, if any, testing or evaluation might be right for you.

IN CONCLUSION . . .

Wow, who knew we could talk so much about vulvas and vaginas and periods and sex and birth control and shame and more?!

(OK, I did, because I literally do this for a living.)

I hope you found whatever it is you needed from this book.

Maybe it was the reassurance that your body is normal. Or maybe you needed permission to ask for help or talk to your doctor or tell your partner who isn't treating you right that you aren't going to take it anymore.

My only ask now that you've read this is that you pass it along. Not only the information you've learned in this book, but the overall rejection of shame culture when it comes to body image and sexual health.

Use your power by not purchasing products that make a profit by making you feel dirty. Unfollow the accounts on social media that peddle misinformation and hype and fear. Call out the BS when you see it.

Most importantly: speak up. You are worth it. You deserve to be seen and heard. If you don't feel you are getting that from your doctor, find a second or third or fourth opinion.

The personal messages I have gotten from my followers are the reason this book is here today. When you tell me that you've finally accepted your body or felt empowered to advocate for yourself because of my posts—it has made my work worth it.

All right, good chat!

ACKNOWLEDGMENTS

This book wouldn't be here without the many people (mostly women!) who believed in and supported me along the way:

To Willi Galloway, for thinking my social media posts about vulvas and vaginal discharge might make an interesting book and for introducing me to your book agent. I am so thankful for you and everyone in our fabulous book club.

To Joy Tutela at the David Black Literary Agency, and said literary agent, who believed in this idea and worked so hard to bring my book to fruition. I've been so lucky to have you in my corner, teaching me the ways of this business!

To my editor, Allison Adler, and the entire team at Andrews McMeel Publishing, who took a chance on a new author in the middle of a pandemic. Thank you so much for all your hard work and for tolerating my obsession over fonts and colors.

To Charlotte Willcox, my amazing illustrator, who brought my words to life in a realistic way so everyone can see themselves in this book. I can't wait to fly across the pond and meet you in person one day!

To my mom, who when I was in elementary school brought me to the library so I could look up publishing house addresses to submit a story I had written. They rejected me, but your belief in what I could do gave me the confidence to keep going.

To my dad, who, like my mom, always knew I could do whatever I wanted if I worked hard enough. Yes, Dad, I double-checked my work (so did the copyeditors).

To my social media doctor besties who have given me more support over a screen than I thought possible: Your confidence in what we are doing to help patients is why I jumped in in the first place. Thank you.

To Dr. Maureen Baldwin, Dr. Suzanne Burlone, Dr. Kara Connelly, Dr. Abby Furukawa, Dr. Anu Kathiresan, Dr. Staci Tanouye, and Dr. Simone van Swam: Thank you for reviewing my book and for your amazingly insightful suggestions. This book is infinitely better because of your input. I have such badass friends.

To the patients I have cared for: I am privileged to be able to do what I do every day, and I am honored by the trust you place in me. You have all taught me so very much.

To those who have trained me and those I get to work with every day, thank you for your ongoing support. Nothing will ever top what we get to do every day at work, and I am so privileged to have learned from and work with such a talented group of people so dedicated to caring for women.

To those of you who have reached out on social media and shared stories of how my posts gave you the confidence to speak up, seek care, and feel comfortable in your body: I read every one of those messages, and I thank you so very deeply.

To my husband, who is married to a vagina doctor and could roll his eyes with my social media presence but instead brags about it and keeps me going when I feel down: Thank you for always believing in me. Good thing I said yes to that friendly dinner back in 2003.

And to my two sons, who have no idea what my book is really about but definitely will one day, know that I am always here for you and no conversation is too embarrassing to have. Your open-minded generation gives me so much hope. I love you both.

REFERENCES

Period Puzzles

Why is my period heavy and making me miserable?
American College of Obstetricians and Gynecologists. "Diagnosis of Abnormal Uterine Bleeding in Reproductive-Aged Women" (July 2012). https://www.acog.org/clinical/clinical-guidance/practice-bulletin/articles/2012/07/diagnosis-of-abnormal-uterine-bleeding-in-reproductive-aged-women.

ACOG. "Dysmenorrhea and Endometriosis in the Adolescent" (December 2018). https://www.acog.org/clinical/clinical-guidance/committee-opinion/articles/2018/12/dysmenorrhea-and-endometriosis-in-the-adolescent.

ACOG. "Dysmenorrhea: Painful Periods." Accessed June 2020. https://www.acog.org/patient-resources/faqs/gynecologic-problems/dysmenorrhea-painful-periods.

ACOG. "Management of Acute Abnormal Uterine Bleeding in Nonpregnant Reproductive-Aged Women" (April 2013). https://www.acog.org/clinical/clinical-guidance/committee-opinion/articles/2013/04/management-of-acute-abnormal-uterine-bleeding-in-nonpregnant-reproductive-aged-women.

What does it mean if I'm bleeding in between my periods?
American College of Obstetricians and Gynecologists. "Diagnosis of Abnormal Uterine Bleeding in Reproductive-Aged Women" (July 2012). https://www.acog.org/clinical/clinical-guidance/practice-bulletin/articles/2012/07/diagnosis-of-abnormal-uterine-bleeding-in-reproductive-aged-women.

I only have a few periods a year—is that OK?

American College of Obstetricians and Gynecologists. "Diagnosis of Abnormal Uterine Bleeding in Reproductive-Aged Women" (July 2012). https://www.acog.org/clinical/clinical-guidance/practice-bulletin/articles/2012/07/diagnosis-of-abnormal-uterine-bleeding-in-reproductive-aged-women.

ACOG. "Infertility Workup for the Women's Health Specialist" (June 2010). https://www.acog.org/clinical/clinical-guidance/committee-opinion/articles/2019/06/infertility-workup-for-the-womens-health-specialist.

ACOG. "Primary Ovarian Insufficiency in Adolescents and Young Women" (July 2014). https://www.acog.org/clinical/clinical-guidance/committee-opinion/articles/2014/07/primary-ovarian-insufficiency-in-adolescents-and-young-women.

Can I get pregnant on my period?

American Society for Reproductive Medicine. "Optimizing Natural Fertility: A Committee Opinion" (January 2017). https://www.asrm.org/globalassets/asrm/asrm-content/news-and-publications/practice-guidelines/for-non-members/optimizing_natural_fertility.pdf.

I've heard periods are supposed to hurt. Is this true?

American College of Obstetricians and Gynecologists. "Diagnosis of Abnormal Uterine Bleeding in Reproductive-Aged Women" (July 2012). https://www.acog.org/clinical/clinical-guidance/practice-bulletin/articles/2012/07/diagnosis-of-abnormal-uterine-bleeding-in-reproductive-aged-women.

ACOG. "Dysmenorrhea and Endometriosis in the Adolescent" (December 2018). https://www.acog.org/clinical/clinical-guidance/committee-opinion/articles/2018/12/dysmenorrhea-and-endometriosis-in-the-adolescent.

Do I need organic tampons?
DeVito, Michael J. and Arnold Schecter. "Exposure Assessment to Dioxins from the Use of Tampons and Diapers." *Environmental Health Perspectives* 110, no. 1 (January 2002): 23-28. https://www.ncbi.nlm.nih.gov/pmc/articles/PMC1240689/.

Mikkelson, David. "Asbestos in Tampons." Snopes. Accessed June 2020. https://www.snopes.com/fact-check/asbestos-in-tampons.

Nonfoux, Louis et al. "Impact of Currently Marketed Tampons and Menstrual Cups on *Staphylococcus aureus* Growth and Toxic Shock Syndrome Toxic 1 Production *In Vitro*." American Society for Microbiology (May 2018). https://aem.asm.org/content/84/12/e00351-18.full#sec-9.

Are menstrual cups OK?
Long, Jill et al. "Menstrual Cup Use and Intrauterine Device Expulsion in a Copper Intrauterine Device Contraceptive Efficacy Trial." *Obstetrics & Gynecology* (May 2020). https://journals.lww.com/greenjournal/pages/articleviewer.aspx?year=2020&issue=05001&article=00003&type=Abstract.

van Eijk, Anna Maria et al. "Menstrual Cup Use, Leakage, Acceptability, Safety, and Availability: A Systemic Review and Meta-analysis." *Lancet Public Health* 4 (July 16, 2019): e361-93. https://www.thelancet.com/journals/lanpub/article/PIIS2468-2667(19)30111-2.

Are period underwear gross?
VanLeeuwen, Crystal and Belen Torondel. "Exploring Menstrual Practices and Potential Accessibility of Reusable Menstrual Underwear among a Middle Eastern Population Living in a Refugee Setting." *International Journal of Women's Health* 10 (July 12, 2018): 349-360. https://www.ncbi.nlm.nih.gov/pmc/articles/PMC6047600.

Is PMDD a real thing?
MGH Center for Women's Mental Health. "PMS and PMDD." Accessed May 15, 2020. https://womensmentalhealth.org/posts/category/pms-and-pmdd.

Thielen, Jacqueline M. "Premenstrual Dysphoric Disorder: Different from PMS?" Mayo Clinic (November 29, 2018). https://www.mayoclinic.org/diseases-conditions/premenstrual-syndrome/expert-answers/pmdd/faq-20058315.

Care and Curiosities for Down There

Why am I always wet?
American College of Obstetricians and Gynecologists. "Vaginitis in Nonpregnant Patients" (January 2020). https://www.acog.org/clinical/clinical-guidance/practice-bulletin/articles/2020/01/vaginitis-in-nonpregnant-patients.

Mayo Clinic Staff. "Vaginal Discharge: Definition." Mayo Clinic. Accessed July 2020. https://www.mayoclinic.org/symptoms/vaginal-discharge/basics/definition/sym-20050825.

Merriam-Webster. "Physiological." Accessed July 2020. https://www.merriam-webster.com/dictionary/physiological.

What does normal vaginal discharge look like?
American College of Obstetricians and Gynecologists. "Fertility Awareness-Based Methods of Family Planning" (January 2019). https://www.acog.org/patient-resources/faqs/contraception/fertility-awareness-based-methods-of-family-planning.

ACOG. "Vaginitis in Nonpregnant Patients" (January 2020). https://www.acog.org/clinical/clinical-guidance/practice-bulletin/articles/2020/01/vaginitis-in-nonpregnant-patients.

American Society for Reproductive Medicine. "Optimizing Natural Fertility: A Committee Opinion" (January 2017). https://www.asrm.org/globalassets/asrm/asrm-content/news-and-publications/practice-guidelines/for-non-members/optimizing_natural_fertility.pdf.

Planned Parenthood. "What's the Cervical Mucus Method of FAMs?" Accessed July 2020. https://www.plannedparenthood.org/learn/birth-control/fertility-awareness/whats-cervical-mucus-method-fams.

How do I know if there's a problem with my discharge?
American College of Obstetricians and Gynecologists. "Vaginitis in Nonpregnant Patients" (January 2020). https://www.acog.org/clinical/clinical-guidance/practice-bulletin/articles/2020/01/vaginitis-in-nonpregnant-patients.

Nyirjesy, Paul et al. "Causes of Chronic Vaginitis: Analysis of a Prospective Database of Affected Women." *Obstetrics & Gynecology* 108, no. 5 (November 2006): 1185-91. https://pubmed.ncbi.nlm.nih.gov/17077241.

What soap is best to clean my vagina?
American College of Obstetricians and Gynecologists. "Vulvovaginal Health" (January 2020). https://www.acog.org/patient-resources/faqs/womens-health/vulvovaginal-health.

Gunter, Jen. "How Should I Be Washing My Vulva on a Day-to-Day Basis?" Accessed July 2020. https://www.nytimes.com/ask/answers/how-should-i-be-washing-my-vulva-day-to-day.

Can I douche?
Martino, Jenny L. and Sten H. Vermund. "Vaginal Douching: Evidence for Risks or Benefits to Women's Health." *Epidemiology Reviews* 24, no. 2 (2002): 109-124. https://www.ncbi.nlm.nih.gov/pmc/articles/PMC2567125.

Office on Women's Health. "Douching." U.S. Department of Health & Human Services. Accessed July 2020. https://www.womenshealth.gov/a-z-topics/douching.

How do I fix the pH of my vagina?

American College of Obstetricians and Gynecologists. "Vaginitis in Nonpregnant Patients" (January 2020). https://www.acog.org/clinical/clinical-guidance/practice-bulletin/articles/2020/01/vaginitis-in-nonpregnant-patients.

Can steaming help my vagina?

Robert, Magali. "Second-Degree Burn Sustained After Vaginal Steaming." *Journal of Obstetrics and Gynecology Canada* 41, no. 6 (2018): 838-839. https://www.clinicalkey.com/#!/content/playContent/1-s2.0-S1701216318305875.

Vandenburg, Tycho and Virginia Braun. "'Basically, It's Sorcery for Your Vagina': Unpacking Western Representations of Vaginal Steaming." *Culture, Health & Sexuality* 19, no. 4 (2017): 470-485. https://www.tandfonline.com/doi/full/10.1080/13691058.2016.1237674.

Wellness Letter. "Ask the Experts: Is Vaginal Steaming Ever a 'Do'?" Berkeley Wellness (February 2020). https://www.berkeleywellness.com/self-care/sexual-health/article/vaginal-steaming-ever-do.

Yoni eggs and yoni pearls: yay or nay?

Carazas, Andrea. "Yoni Pearls: Everything You Need to Know." Mount Sinai Adolescent Health Center (May 2020). https://www.teenhealthcare.org/blog/yoni-pearls.

Gunter, Jennifer. "Dear Gwyneth Paltrow, I'm a GYN and your vaginal jade eggs are a bad idea." *Dr. Jen Gunter* (January 2017). https://drjengunter.com/2017/01/17/dear-gwyneth-paltrow-im-a-gyn-and-your-vaginal-jade-eggs-are-a-bad-idea.

Gunter, Jennifer and Sarah Parcak. "Vaginal Jade Eggs: Ancient Chinese Practice or Modern Marketing Myth?" *Female Pelvic Medicine & Reconstructive Surgery* 25, no. 1 (January/February 2019): 1-2. https://pubmed.ncbi.nlm.nih.gov/30365448.

What is the best way to remove my pubic hair?
American Academy of Dermatology Association. "Laser Hair Removal: FAQs." Accessed July 2020. https://www.aad.org/public/cosmetic/hair-removal/laser-hair-removal-faqs.

Engel, Meredith. "Experts Warn Against Using Depilatories Like Veet, Nair." *New York Daily News* (March 10, 2015). https://www.nydailynews.com/lifestyle/health/experts-warn-depilatories-veet-nair-article-1.2144447.

Leonard, Jayne. "What You Should Know About Laser Hair Removal Versus Electrolysis." *Medical News Today* (December 16, 2017). https://www.medicalnewstoday.com/articles/320329.

Olsen, Elise A. "Methods of Hair Removal." *Journal of the American Academy of Dermatology* 40, no. 2 (February 1, 1999): 143-155. https://www.jaad.org/article/S0190-9622(99)70181-7/fulltext.

My partner says my vagina smells funny—what could it be?
American College of Obstetricians and Gynecologists. "FAQ 190: Vulvovaginal Health" (January 2020). https://www.acog.org/Patients/FAQs/Vulvovaginal-Health.

Miller, Robyn R., M.D. "Vaginal Discharge: What's Normal, What's Not." TeensHealth from Nemours (October 2018). https://kidshealth.org/en/teens/vdischarge2.html.

Office of Population Affairs. "Reproductive Health." U.S. Department of Health & Human Services. Accessed July 2020. https://opa.hhs.gov/reproductive-health.

Should I take probiotics to keep my vagina healthy?
Harvard Women's Health Watch. "Does Your Vagina Really Need a Probiotic?" Harvard Health Publishing (July 2019). https://www.health.harvard.edu/womens-health/does-your-vagina-really-need-a-probiotic.

National Center for Complementary and Integrative Health. "Probiotics: What You Need to Know." National Institutes of Health. Accessed July 2020. https://www.nccih.nih.gov/health/probiotics-what-you-need-to-know.

Senok, Abiola C. et al. "Probiotics for the Treatment of Bacterial Vaginosis." Cochrane Library (July 2009). https://www.cochranelibrary.com/cdsr/doi/10.1002/14651858.CD006289.

Wang, Ziyue, Yining He, and Yingjie Zheng. "Probiotics for Treatment of Bacterial Vaginosis: A Meta-Analysis." *International Journal of Environmental Research and Public Health* 16, no. 20 (October 2019): 3859. https://www.ncbi.nlm.nih.gov/pmc/articles/PMC6848925.

Xie, Huan Yu et al. "Probiotics for Vulvovaginal Candidiasis in Non-pregnant Women." Cochrane Library (November 2017). https://www.cochranelibrary.com/cdsr/doi/10.1002/14651858.CD010496.

How do I know if my labia are normal?

The Labia Library. "Have You Ever Wondered 'Is My Vagina Normal?' Lots of Women Have." Women's Health Victoria. Accessed July 2020. http://www.labialibrary.org.au.

Can I lighten my labia?

The American College of Obstetricians and Gynecologists. "Vulvovaginal Health Pamphlet" (February 2020). https://www.acog.org/store/products/patient-education/pamphlets/womens-health/vulvovaginal-health.

Can I ask my doctor to shorten my labia?

American College of Obstetricians and Gynecologists. "Elective Female Genital Cosmetic Surgery" (January 2020). https://www.acog.org/clinical/clinical-guidance/committee-opinion/articles/2020/01/elective-female-genital-cosmetic-surgery.

How do I tighten my vagina?

American College of Obstetricians and Gynecologists. "Elective Female Genital Cosmetic Surgery" (January 2020). https://www.acog.org/clinical/clinical-guidance/committee-opinion/articles/2020/01/elective-female-genital-cosmetic-surgery.

ACOG. "Female Sexual Dysfunction" (July 2019). https://www.acog.org/clinical/clinical-guidance/practice-bulletin/articles/2019/07/female-sexual-dysfunction.

ACOG. "Pelvic Support Problems" (October 2017). https://www.acog.org/patient-resources/faqs/gynecologic-problems/pelvic-support-problems.

U.S. Food and Drug Administration. "FDA Warns Against Use of Energy-Based Devices to Perform Vaginal 'Rejuvenation' or Vaginal Cosmetic Procedures: FDA Safety Communication" (July 30, 2018). https://www.fda.gov/medical-devices/safety-communications/fda-warns-against-use-energy-based-devices-perform-vaginal-rejuvenation-or-vaginal-cosmetic.

Is it normal to leak urine sometimes?

American College of Obstetricians and Gynecologists. "Urinary Incontinence" (August 2019). https://www.acog.org/patient-resources/faqs/gynecologic-problems/urinary-incontinence.

American College of Obstetricians and Gynecologists. "Urinary Incontinence in Women" (November 2015). https://www.acog.org/clinical/clinical-guidance/practice-bulletin/articles/2015/11/urinary-incontinence-in-women.

Facts for Feeling Good

If sex and putting in tampons hurt, what do I do?

American College of Obstetricians and Gynecologists. "Female Sexual Dysfunction" (July 2019). https://www.acog.org/clinical/clinical-guidance/practice-bulletin/articles/2019/07/female-sexual-dysfunction.

ACOG. "When Sex Is Painful" (September 2017). https://www.acog.org/patient-resources/faqs/gynecologic-problems/when-sex-is-painful.

How do I clean a dildo?
American College of Obstetricians and Gynecologists. "Addressing Health Risks of Noncoital Sexual Activity" (December 2013). https://www.acog.org/clinical/clinical-guidance/committee-opinion/articles/2013/12/addressing-health-risks-of-noncoital-sexual-activity.

Planned Parenthood. "Sex Toys" Accessed July 2020. https://www.plannedparenthood.org/learn/sex-pleasure-and-sexual-dysfunction/sex-and-pleasure/sex-toys.

Rubin, Elizabeth S. et al. "A Clinical Reference Guide on Sexual Devices for Obstetrician–Gynecologists." *Obstetrics & Gynecology* 133, no. 6 (June 2019): 1259-1268. https://journals.lww.com/greenjournal/Fulltext/2019/06000/A_Clinical_Reference_Guide_on_Sexual_Devices_for.26.

What lubes are OK to use?
American College of Obstetricians and Gynecologists. "Vulvovaginal Health" (February 2020). https://www.acog.org/store/products/patient-education/pamphlets/womens-health/vulvovaginal-health.

International Society for Sexual Medicine. "What Is a Lubricant?" Accessed July 2020. https://www.issm.info/sexual-health-qa/what-is-a-lubricant.

Where is my G-spot?
American College of Obstetricians and Gynecologists. "Elective Female Genital Cosmetic Surgery" (January 2020). https://www.acog.org/clinical/clinical-guidance/committee-opinion/articles/2020/01/elective-female-genital-cosmetic-surgery.

Kilchevsky, Amichai et al. "Is the Female G-Spot Truly a Distinct Anatomic Entity?" *The Journal of Sexual Medicine* 9, no. 3 (March 2012): 719-726. https://www.sciencedirect.com/science/article/abs/pii/S1743609515338820.

Will I bleed the first time I have sex?

American College of Obstetricians and Gynecologists. "Diagnosis and Management of Hymenal Variants" (June 2019). https://www.acog.org/clinical/clinical-guidance/committee-opinion/articles/2019/06/diagnosis-and-management-of-hymenal-variants.

UK National Health Service. "Does a Woman Always Bleed When She Has Sex for the First Time?" (August 20, 2018). https://www.nhs.uk/common-health-questions/sexual-health/does-a-woman-always-bleed-when-she-has-sex-for-the-first-time.

Do over-the-counter libido supplements really work?

American College of Obstetricians and Gynecologists. "Female Sexual Dysfunction." *Obstetrics & Gynecology* 134, no. 1 (July 2019): e1-e18. https://journals.lww.com/greenjournal/Abstract/2019/07000/Female_Sexual_Dysfunction__ACOG_Practice_Bulletin.45.

Corazza, Ornella et al. "Sexual Enhancement Products for Sale Online: Raising Awareness of the Psychoactive Effects of Yohimbine, Maca, Horny Goat Weed, and *Ginkgo biloba*." *BioMed Research International* (2014): 841798. https://www.ncbi.nlm.nih.gov/pmc/articles/PMC4082836.

Harvard Health Publishing. "Can Supplements Save Your Sex Life?" (February 2019). https://www.health.harvard.edu/staying-healthy/can-supplements-save-your-sex-life.

Is anal sex bad for me?

American College of Obstetricians and Gynecologists. "Addressing Health Risks of Noncoital Sexual Activity" (December 2013). https://www.acog.org/clinical/clinical-guidance/committee-opinion/articles/2013/12/addressing-health-risks-of-noncoital-sexual-activity.

Attia. "Can Anal Sex Have Any Long Term Effects on My Body?" Planned Parenthood (April 2020). https://www.plannedparenthood.org/learn/teens/ ask-experts/can-anal-sex-have-any-long-term-effects-on-my-body-ive-heard- that-it-can-cause-anal-leakage-later-in-life-and-anal-prolapse-is-this-true.

Greer, Tyler. "Anal Sex Linked to Increased Risk of Incontinence in Both Males, Females." Medical Xpress (February 11, 2016). https://medicalxpress.com/ news/2016-02-anal-sex-linked-incontinence-males.html.

UK National Health Service. "Does Anal Sex Have Any Health Risks?" (August 10, 2018). https://www.nhs.uk/common-health-questions/sexual-health/does- anal-sex-have-any-health-risks.

Itching and Burning

Is it OK to use drugstore medicines to treat my yeast infection?

American College of Obstetricians and Gynecologists. "Vaginitis in Nonpregnant Patients" (January 2020). https://www.acog.org/clinical/clinical- guidance/practice-bulletin/articles/2020/01/vaginitis-in-nonpregnant-patients.

Brody, Jane E. "Personal Health; Yeast Infection: The Pitfalls of Self-Diagnosis." *New York Times* (March 19, 2002). https://www.nytimes.com/2002/03/19/ health/personal-health-yeast-infection-the-pitfalls-of-self-diagnosis.html.

Nyirjesy, Paul. "Management of Persistent Vaginitis." *Obstetrics & Gynecology* 124, no. 6 (December 2014): 1135-46. https://pubmed.ncbi.nlm.nih. gov/25415165.

Should I avoid sugar if I'm prone to yeast infections?

Richards, Lisa. "The Candida Diet." Accessed August 2020. https://www. thecandidadiet.com.

Xie, Huan Yu et al. "Probiotics for Vulvovaginal Candidiasis in Non-pregnant Women." Cochrane Library (November 2017). https://www.cochranelibrary. com/cdsr/doi/10.1002/14651858.CD010496.

Why do my yeast infections keep coming back?
American College of Obstetricians and Gynecologists. "Vaginitis in Nonpregnant Patients" (January 2020). https://www.acog.org/clinical/clinical-guidance/practice-bulletin/articles/2020/01/vaginitis-in-nonpregnant-patients.

Aminzadeh, Atousa. "Frequency of Candidiasis and Colonization of *Candida albicans* in Relation to Oral Contraceptive Pills." *Iranian Red Crescent Medical Journal* 18, no. 10 (October 2016): e38909. https://www.ncbi.nlm.nih.gov/pmc/articles/PMC5291939.

Spinillo, A. et al. "The Impact of Oral Contraception on Vulvovaginal Candidiasis." *Contraception* 51, no. 5 (May 1995): 293-7. https://pubmed.ncbi.nlm.nih.gov/7628203.

Boric acid suppositories—do they work?
American College of Obstetricians and Gynecologists. "Vaginitis in Nonpregnant Patients" (January 2020). https://www.acog.org/clinical/clinical-guidance/practice-bulletin/articles/2020/01/vaginitis-in-nonpregnant-patients.

Centers for Disease Control and Prevention. "2015 Sexually Transmitted Diseases Guidelines: Bacterial Vaginosis" (June 4, 2015). https://www.cdc.gov/std/tg2015/bv.htm.

CDC. "2015 Sexually Transmitted Diseases Guidelines: References" (June 4, 2015). https://www.cdc.gov/std/tg2015/references.htm.

Will garlic cure a yeast infection?
Calderone, Julia. "Fact or Fiction?: A Clove of Garlic Can Stop a Vaginal Yeast Infection." *Scientific American* (October 3, 2014). https://www.scientificamerican.com/article/fact-or-fiction-a-clove-of-garlic-can-stop-a-vaginal-yeast-infection.

Cohain, Judy Slome. "How to Treat a Vaginal Infection with a Clove of Garlic." *Midwifery Today* (April 2007). https://midwiferytoday.com/mt-articles/garlic.

Li, Wen-Ru et al. "Antifungal Activity, Kinetics and Molecular Mechanism of Action of Garlic Oil Against *Candida albicans*." *Scientific Reports* 6 (2016): 22805. https://www.ncbi.nlm.nih.gov/pmc/articles/PMC4779998.

Watson, C. J. et al. "The Effects of Oral Garlic on Vaginal Candida Colony Counts: A Randomised Placebo Controlled Double-Blind Trial." *BJOG* 121, no. 4 (March 2014): 498-506. https://pubmed.ncbi.nlm.nih.gov/24308540.

Is bacterial vaginosis an STI?
American College of Obstetricians and Gynecologists. "Vaginitis in Nonpregnant Patients" (January 2020). https://www.acog.org/clinical/clinical-guidance/practice-bulletin/articles/2020/01/vaginitis-in-nonpregnant-patients.

Centers for Disease Control and Prevention. "Bacterial Vaginosis—CDC Fact Sheet" (February 10, 2020). https://www.cdc.gov/std/bv/stdfact-bacterial-vaginosis.htm.

My BV infections won't go away—what do I do?
American College of Obstetricians and Gynecologists. "Vaginitis in Nonpregnant Patients" (January 2020). https://www.acog.org/clinical/clinical-guidance/practice-bulletin/articles/2020/01/vaginitis-in-nonpregnant-patients.

Centers for Disease Control and Prevention. "2015 Sexually Transmitted Diseases Treatment Guidelines: Bacterial Vaginosis" (June 4, 2015). https://www.cdc.gov/std/tg2015/bv.htm.

How do I know if I have an STI?
American College of Obstetricians and Gynecologists. "Chlamydia, Gonorrhea, and Syphilis" (February 2019). https://www.acog.org/womens-health/faqs/chlamydia-gonorrhea-and-syphilis.

ACOG. "Genital Herpes" (June 2019). https://www.acog.org/womens-health/faqs/genital-herpes.

ACOG. "Protecting Yourself Against Hepatitis B and C" (December 2016). https://www.acog.org/womens-health/faqs/protecting-yourself-against-hepatitis-b-and-hepatitis-c.

Mayo Clinic Staff. "Sexually Transmitted Diseases (STDs)." Mayo Clinic (March 13, 2018). https://www.mayoclinic.org/diseases-conditions/sexually-transmitted-diseases-stds/symptoms-causes/syc-20351240.

When I ask for STI testing, what does my doctor order?

Centers for Disease Control and Prevention. "2015 Sexually Transmitted Diseases Treatment Guidelines: Screening Recommendations and Considerations Referenced in Treatment Guidelines and Original Sources" (June 14, 2015). https://www.cdc.gov/std/tg2015/screening-recommendations.htm.

U.S. Preventive Services Task Force. "Genital Herpes Infection: Serologic Screening" (December 20, 2016). https://www.uspreventiveservicestaskforce.org/uspstf/recommendation/genital-herpes-screening.

I have chlamydia, but I don't want to tell my partner. . . . Do I have to?

American College of Obstetricians and Gynecologists. "Expedited Partner Therapy" (June 2018). https://www.acog.org/clinical/clinical-guidance/committee-opinion/articles/2018/06/expedited-partner-therapy.

Can lesbians get STIs too?

American College of Obstetricians and Gynecologists. "Health Care for Lesbians and Bisexual Women" (May 2012). https://www.acog.org/clinical/clinical-guidance/committee-opinion/articles/2012/05/health-care-for-lesbians-and-bisexual-women.

Mayo Clinic Staff. "Health Issues for Lesbians and Women Who Have Sex with Women." Mayo Clinic (October 10, 2017). https://www.mayoclinic.org/healthy-lifestyle/adult-health/in-depth/health-issues-for-lesbians/art-20047202.

Mravcak, Sally A. "Primary Care for Lesbians and Bisexual Women." *American Family Physician* 74, no. 2 (July 15, 2006): 279-286. https://www.aafp.org/afp/2006/0715/p279.html.

WebMD. "Dental Dam" (June 27, 2020). https://www.webmd.com/hiv-aids/dental-dam-how-to-use.

Do I have to tell my partner that I get cold sores?

Centers for Disease Control and Prevention. "Genital Herpes—CDC Fact Sheet" (August 28, 2017). https://www.cdc.gov/std/herpes/stdfact-herpes.htm.

McQuillan, Geraldine et al. "Prevalence of Herpes Simplex Virus Type 1 and Type 2 in Persons Aged 14–49: United States, 2015-2016." *NCHS Data Brief No. 304* (February 2018). https://www.cdc.gov/nchs/products/databriefs/db304.htm.

Can I contract an infection just from oral sex?

American College of Obstetricians and Gynecologists. "Addressing Health Risks of Noncoital Sexual Activity" (December 2013). https://www.acog.org/clinical/clinical-guidance/committee-opinion/articles/2013/12/addressing-health-risks-of-noncoital-sexual-activity.

Centers for Disease Control and Prevention. "STD Risk and Oral Sex—CDC Fact Sheet" (February 27, 2020). https://www.cdc.gov/std/healthcomm/stdfact-stdriskandoralsex.htm.

Dahlstrom, Kristina R. et al. "Differences in History of Sexual Behavior Between Patients with Oropharyngeal Squamous Cell Carcinoma and Patients with Squamous Cell Carcinoma at Other Head and Neck Sites." *Head & Neck* 33, no. 6 (June 2011): 847-855. https://www.ncbi.nlm.nih.gov/pmc/articles/PMC2994955.

Edwards, Sarah and Chris Carne. "Oral Sex and the Transmission of Non-viral STIs." *Sexually Transmitted Infections* 74 (1998): 95-100. https://www.ncbi.nlm.nih.gov/pmc/articles/PMC1758102/pdf/v074p00095.pdf.

Holway, Giuseppina Valle and Stephanie M. Hernandez. "Oral Sex and Condom Use in a U.S. National Sample of Adolescents and Young Adults." *Journal of Adolescent Health* 62, no. 4 (April 2018): 402-410. https://pubmed.ncbi.nlm.nih.gov/29174873.

Which STIs are curable . . . and which ones aren't?
Centers for Disease Control and Prevention. "2015 Sexually Transmitted Diseases Treatment Guidelines: Summary" Accessed August 2020. https://www.cdc.gov/std/tg2015/default.htm.

When does chlamydia turn into PID and cause infertility?
American College of Obstetricians and Gynecologists. "Pelvic Inflammatory Disease (PID)" (August 2019). https://www.acog.org/patient-resources/faqs/gynecologic-problems/pelvic-inflammatory-disease.

Centers for Disease Control and Prevention. "2015 Sexually Transmitted Diseases Treatment Guidelines: Pelvic Inflammatory Disease (PID)" (June 4, 2015). https://www.cdc.gov/std/tg2015/pid.htm.

Wiesenfeld, Harold C. et al. "Subclinical Pelvic Inflammatory Disease and Infertility." *Obstetrics & Gynecology* 120, no. 1 (July 2012): 37-43. https://pubmed.ncbi.nlm.nih.gov/22678036.

Birth Control Basics

How do I start birth control without my parents knowing?
Dreweke, Joerg. "Promiscuity Propaganda: Access to Information and Services Does Not Lead to Increases in Sexual Activity." *Guttmacher Policy Review* (June 11, 2019). https://www.guttmacher.org/gpr/2019/06/promiscuity-propaganda-access-information-and-services-does-not-lead-increases-sexual.

Guttmacher Institute. "An Overview of Consent to Reproductive Health Services by Young People." Guttmacher Institute. Accessed August 2020. https://www.guttmacher.org/state-policy/explore/overview-minors-consent-law.

Secura, Gina M., Tiffany Adams, and Jeffrey F. Peipert. "Change in Sexual Behavior with Provision of No-Cost Contraception." *Obstetrics & Gynecology* 123, no. 4 (April 2014): 771-776. https://www.ncbi.nlm.nih.gov/pmc/articles/PMC4009508.

Does getting an IUD insertion hurt?
Akdemir, Yesim and Mustafa Karadeniz. "The Relationship Between Pain at IUD Insertion and Negative Perceptions, Anxiety and Previous Mode of Delivery." *The European Journal of Contraception and Reproductive Health Care* 24, no. 3 (May 2019): 1-6. https://www.researchgate.net/publication/333157053.

Allen, Rebecca H. et al. "Interventions for Pain with Intrauterine Device Insertion." Cochrane Library (October 8, 2008). https://doi.org/10.1002/14651858.CD007373.

Can I use an IUD if I haven't had a baby?
American College of Obstetricians and Gynecologists. "Adolescents and Long-Acting Reversible Contraception: Implants and Intrauterine Devices" (May 2018). https://www.acog.org/clinical/clinical-guidance/committee-opinion/articles/2018/05/adolescents-and-long-acting-reversible-contraception-implants-and-intrauterine-devices.

ACOG. "Long-Acting Reversible Contraception: Implants and Intrauterine Devices" (November 2017). https://www.acog.org/clinical/clinical-guidance/practice-bulletin/articles/2017/11/long-acting-reversible-contraception-implants-and-intrauterine-devices.

Do antibiotics mess with birth control?
Amy. "Is It True That Antibiotics Can Make Birth Control Stop Working?" Planned Parenthood (October, 14, 2010). https://www.plannedparenthood.org/learn/teens/ask-experts/i-was-watching-tv-and-they-said-that-if-your-on-birth-control-and-taking-antibiotics-the-birth-control-will-stop-working-im-on-the-pill-right-now-and-ive-had-to-start-taking-antibiotics-because-o.

Archer, Johanna S. M. and David F. Archer. "Oral Contraceptive Efficacy and Antibiotic Interaction: A Myth Debunked." *Am Acad Dermatol.* 46, no. 6 (June 2002): 917-23. doi: 10.1067/mjd.2002.120448. https://pubmed.ncbi.nlm.nih.gov/12063491/.

Aronson, Jeffrey K. and Robin E. Ferner. "Analysis of Reports of Unintended Pregnancies Associated with the Combined Use of Non-Enzyme-Inducing Antibiotics and Hormonal Contraceptives." *BMJ Evidence-Based Medicine* (2020). https://ebm.bmj.com/content/early/2020/07/28/bmjebm-2020-111363.

DeRossi, Scott S. and Elliot V. Hersh. "Antibiotics and Oral Contraceptives." *Dent Clin North Am.* 46, no. 4 (October 2002): 653-64. doi: 10.1016/s0011-8532(02)00017-4. PMID: 12436822. https://pubmed.ncbi.nlm.nih.gov/12436822/.

Zhanel, G. G. et al. "Antibiotic and Oral Contraceptive Drug Interactions: Is There a Need for Concern?" *Can J Infect Dis.* 10, no. 6 (November 1999): 429-33. doi: 10.1155/1999/539376. https://pubmed.ncbi.nlm.nih.gov/22346401/.

Does melatonin "cancel out" my birth control?

Flynn, Caitlin. "If You're on the Pill and You Regularly Take Melatonin, Read This Important Warning." *POPSUGAR* (July 30, 2020). https://www.popsugar.com/fitness/Does-Melatonin-Make-Your-Birth-Control-Less-Effective-46359481.

Mayo Clinic Staff. "Melatonin." Mayo Clinic (March 30, 2018). https://www.mayoclinic.org/drugs-supplements-melatonin/art-20363071.

Peuhkuri, Katri, Nora Sihvola, and Riitta Korpela. "Dietary Factors and Fluctuating Levels of Melatonin." *Food & Nutrition Research* 56 (2012). https://www.ncbi.nlm.nih.gov/pmc/articles/PMC3402070.

Do I have to take my pill the same time every day?
Curtis, Kathryn M. et al. "U.S. Selected Practice Recommendations for Contraceptive Use, 2016." Centers for Disease Control and Prevention, *Recommendations and Reports* 65, no. 4 (July 29, 2016): 1-66. https://www.cdc.gov/mmwr/volumes/65/rr/rr6504a1.htm.

Planned Parenthood. "How Do I Use the Birth Control Pill?" Accessed March 13, 2020. https://www.plannedparenthood.org/learn/birth-control/birth-control-pill/how-do-i-use-the-birth-control-pill.

Can I just use condoms?
Aisch, Gregor and Bill Marsh. "How Likely Is It That Birth Control Could Let You Down?" *New York Times* (September 13, 2014). https://www.nytimes.com/interactive/2014/09/14/sunday-review/unplanned-pregnancies.html.

Bedsider. "Condom." Accessed March 14, 2020. https://www.bedsider.org/methods/condom.

Centers for Disease Control and Prevention. "Male Condom Use" (July 6, 2016). https://www.cdc.gov/condomeffectiveness/male-condom-use.html.

How do I know if a condom is OK to use?
Bedsider. "Condom." Accessed March 14, 2020. https://www.bedsider.org/methods/condom.

Bedsider. "How Do I Check a Condom Wrapper for Damage?" Accessed March 14, 2020. https://www.bedsider.org/questions/306-how-do-i-check-a-condom-wrapper-for-damage.

Will birth control make it harder to become pregnant when I'm older?
International Planned Parenthood Federation. "Myths and Facts about . . . the Contraceptive Pill" (March 11, 2019). https://www.ippf.org/blogs/myths-and-facts-about-contraceptive-pill.

Mansour, Diana et al. "Fertility after Discontinuation of Contraception: A Comprehensive Review of the Literature." *Contraception* 84, no. 5 (November 2011): https://pubmed.ncbi.nlm.nih.gov/22018120.

Which birth control will make me gain weight?

American College of Obstetricians and Gynecologists. "Progestin-Only Hormonal Birth Control: Pill and Injection" (October 2020). https://www.acog.org/patient-resources/faqs/contraception/progestin-only-hormonal-birth-control-pill-and-injection.

Bonny, Andrea E. et al. "Weight Gain in Obese and Nonobese Adolescent Girls Initiating Depot Medroxyprogestrone, Oral Contraceptive Pills, or No Hormonal Contraceptive Method." *Archives of Pediatrics & Adolescent Medicine* 160, no. 1 (January 2006): 40-5. https://pubmed.ncbi.nlm.nih.gov/16389209.

Chambers, Edward S. et al. "Effects of Targeted Delivery of Propionate to the Human Colon on Appetite Regulation, Body Weight Maintenance and Adiposity in Overweight Adults." *Gut* 64 (2015): 1744-1754. https://gut.bmj.com/content/64/11/1744.

Cochrane Library. "Effect of Birth Control Pills and Patches on Weight" (January 29, 2014). https://www.cochrane.org/CD003987.

Cochrane Library. "Effects of Progestin-Only Birth Control on Weight" (August 28, 2016). https://www.cochrane.org/CD008815.

Institute for Quality and Efficiency in Health Care. "Contraception: Do Hormonal Contraceptives Cause Weight Gain?" (June 29, 2017). https://www.ncbi.nlm.nih.gov/books/NBK441582.

Le, Yen-Chi, Mahbubur Rahman, and Abbey B. Berenson. "Early Weight Gain Predicting Later Weight Gain among Depot Medroxyprogesterone Acetate Users." *Obstetrics & Gynecology* 114, no. 2 (August 2009): 279-284. https://pubmed.ncbi.nlm.nih.gov/19622988.

Wallace, Robin. "Does Birth Control Really Make You Fat?" Bedsider (October 1, 2010). https://www.bedsider.org/features/100-does-birth-control-really-make-you-fat.

Will birth control mess with my sex drive?
Barr, Nancy Grossman. "Managing Adverse Effects of Hormonal Contraceptives." *American Family Physician* 15, no. 82 (December 15, 2010): 1499-1506. https://www.aafp.org/afp/2010/1215/p1499.html.

Boozalis, Amanda, Nhial T. Tutlam, and Jeffrey F. Peipert. "Sexual Desire and Hormonal Contraception." *Obstetrics & Gynecology* 127, no. 3 (March 2016): 563-572. https://www.ncbi.nlm.nih.gov/pmc/articles/PMC4764410.

Can birth control help my acne?
American College of Obstetricians and Gynecologists. "Noncontraceptive Uses of Hormonal Contraceptives" (January 2010). https://www.acog.org/clinical/clinical-guidance/practice-bulletin/articles/2010/01/noncontraceptive-uses-of-hormonal-contraceptives.

Arowojolu, Ayodele O. et al. "Combined Oral Contraceptive Pills for Treatment of Acne." *Cochrane Database System Review* 13, no. 6 (June 13, 2012). https://pubmed.ncbi.nlm.nih.gov/22696343.

Will birth control make me depressed?
Schaffir, Jonathan, Brett L. Worly, and Tamar L. Gur. "Combined Hormonal Contraception and its Effects on Mood: A Critical Review." *European Journal of Controception & Reproductive Health Care* 21, no. 5 (October 2016): 347-55. https://pubmed.ncbi.nlm.nih.gov/27636867.

Skovlund, Charlotte Wessel et al. "Association of Hormonal Contraception with Depression." *JAMA Psychiatry* 73, no. 11 (November 2016): 1154-1162. https://jamanetwork.com/journals/jamapsychiatry/fullarticle/2552796.

What birth control doesn't have any hormones?

Allen, Richard E. "Diaphragm Fitting." *American Family Physician* 69, no. 1 (January 1, 2004): 97-100. https://www.aafp.org/afp/2004/0101/p97.html.

Bedsider. "Method Explorer" Accessed August 2020. https://www.bedsider. org/methods.

CooperSurgical, Inc. "Paragard: Intrauterine Copper Contraceptive" (February 2020). https://www.paragard.com/wp-content/uploads/2018/10/ PARAGARD-PI.pdf.

Evofem, Inc. "Full Prescribing Information: PHEXXI" (May 2020). https://www. phexxi.com/themes/custom/phexxiDTC/dist/pdf/PhexxiUSPI.pdf.

Guttmacher Institute. "Contraceptive Effectiveness in the United States" (April 2020). https://www.guttmacher.org/fact-sheet/contraceptive-effectiveness-united-states.

National Women's Health Network. "Fact Sheet: Phexxi Contraceptive Gel." Accessed August 2020. https://www.nwhn.org/phexxi.

Are online companies that ship birth control legit?

American College of Obstetricians and Gynecologists. "Over-the-Counter Access to Hormonal Contraception" (October 2019). https://www.acog. org/clinical/clinical-guidance/committee-opinion/articles/2019/10/over-the-counter-access-to-hormonal-contraception.

National Alliance of State Pharmacy Associations. "Pharmacist Prescribing: Hormonal Contraceptives" (August 20, 2020). https://naspa.us/resource/ contraceptives.

Rodriguez, Maria I., Lorinda Anderson, and Alison B. Edelman. "Pharmacists Begin Prescribing Hormonal Contraception in Oregon: Implementation of House Bill 2879." *Obstetrics & Gynecology* 128, no. 1 (July 2016): 168-170. https://www.ncbi.nlm.nih.gov/pmc/articles/PMC4917426.

Does alcohol or CBD affect birth control?

Jiang, Rongrong et al. "Identification of Cytochrome P450 Enzymes Responsible for Metabolism of Cannabidiol by Human Liver Microsomes." *Life Sciences* (89 (August 1, 2011): 165-170. https://pubmed.ncbi.nlm.nih.gov/21704641/.

Mayo Clinic Staff. "Combination Birth Control Pills." Mayo Clinic (December 17, 2020). https://www.mayoclinic.org/tests-procedures/combination-birth-control-pills/about/pac-20385282.

Nurx. "What If I Get Sick After Taking My Birth Control Pill?" (October 14, 2016). https://www.nurx.com/blog/what-if-i-get-sick-after-taking-my-birth-control-pill.

Smith, Fay. "CBD Oil and Birth Control." CBD Clinicals (January 1, 2021). https://cbdclinicals.com/cbd-oil-and-birth-control.

Why isn't there a birth control pill for men?!

Alton, Kaylee. "Why Isn't There a Hormonal Birth Control for Men?" Clue. (December 11, 2019). https://helloclue.com/articles/sex/why-isnt-there-a-hormonal-birth-control-for-men.

Revolution Contraceptives. "Vasalgel." Accessed August 2020. https://www.revolutioncontraceptives.com/vasalgel.

Thirumalai, Arthi et al. "Effects of 28 Days of Oral Dimethandrolone Undecanoate in Healthy Men: A Prototype Male Pill." *The Journal of Clinical Endocrinology & Metabolism* 104, no. 23 (February 2019): 423-432. https://academic.oup.com/jcem/article/104/2/423/5105935.

UC Davis Health. "Male Contraception Clinical Trial Launches in Sacramento" (June 22, 2020). https://health.ucdavis.edu/health-news/newsroom/male-contraception-clinical-trial-launches-in-sacramento-/2020/06.

Going to the Doctor

Will my doctor do a pelvic exam at my first visit?
American College of Obstetricians and Gynecologists. "Counseling Adolescents About Contraception" (August 2017). https://www.acog.org/clinical/clinical-guidance/committee-opinion/articles/2017/08/counseling-adolescents-about-contraception.

ACOG. "The Initial Reproductive Health Visit" (May 2014). https://www.acog.org/clinical/clinical-guidance/committee-opinion/articles/2014/05/the-initial-reproductive-health-visit.

Centers for Disease Control and Prevention. "Appendix C: Examinations and Tests Needed Before Initiation of Contraceptive Methods" (February 1, 2017). https://www.cdc.gov/reproductivehealth/contraception/mmwr/spr/appendixc.html.

Can I go to the OB-GYN without telling my parents?
Guttmacher Institute. "An Overview of Consent to Reproductive Health Services by Young People." Accessed August 2020. https://www.guttmacher.org/state-policy/explore/overview-minors-consent-law.

Guttmacher Institute. "Minors' Access to Contraceptive Services." Accessed August 2020. https://www.guttmacher.org/state-policy/explore/minors-access-contraceptive-services.

HealthyChildren.org. "Information for Teens: What You Need to Know About Privacy." American Academy of Pediatrics (September 9, 2010). https://www.healthychildren.org/English/ages-stages/teen/Pages/Information-for-Teens-What-You-Need-to-Know-About-Privacy.aspx.

Can my doctor tell my parents what we talked about?
Guttmacher Institute. "An Overview of Consent to Reproductive Health Services by Young People." Accessed August 2020. https://www.guttmacher.org/state-policy/explore/overview-minors-consent-law.

Guttmacher Institute. "Minors' Access to Contraceptive Services." Accessed August 2020. https://www.guttmacher.org/state-policy/explore/minors-access-contraceptive-services.

HealthyChildren.org. "Information for Teens: What You Need to Know About Privacy." American Academy of Pediatrics (September 9, 2010). https://www.healthychildren.org/English/ages-stages/teen/Pages/Information-for-Teens-What-You-Need-to-Know-About-Privacy.aspx.

Will my doctor be able to tell if I've had sex?
World Health Organization. "Eliminating Virginity Testing: An Interagency Statement" (2018). https://www.who.int/reproductivehealth/publications/eliminating-virginity-testing-interagency-statement/en.

Do I have to get a pap smear?
American College of Obstetricians and Gynecologists "Your First Gynecologic Visit" (March 2019). https://www.acog.org/patient-resources/faqs/especially-for-teens/your-first-gynecologic-visit.

Planned Parenthood. "What Is a Pelvic Exam?" Accessed August 2020. https://www.plannedparenthood.org/learn/health-and-wellness/wellness-visit/what-pelvic-exam.

How long can I go between pap smears?
American College of Obstetricians and Gynecologists. "Cervical Cancer Screening (Update)" (August 2018). https://www.acog.org/clinical/clinical-guidance/practice-advisory/articles/2018/08/cervical-cancer-screening-update.

Do lesbians need pap smears?
American College of Obstetricians and Gynecologists. "Health Care for Lesbians and Bisexual Women" (May 2012). https://www.acog.org/clinical/clinical-guidance/committee-opinion/articles/2012/05/health-care-for-lesbians-and-bisexual-women.

Mravcak, Sally A. "Primary Care for Lesbians and Bisexual women." *American Family Physician* 74, no. 2 (July 15, 2006): 279-286. https://www.aafp.org/afp/2006/0715/p279.html.

Can I ask my doctor to check for a hormone imbalance?
American College of Obstetricians and Gynecologists. "Compounded Bioidentical Menopausal Hormone Therapy" (August 2012). https://www.acog.org/clinical/clinical-guidance/committee-opinion/articles/2012/08/compounded-bioidentical-menopausal-hormone-therapy.

Everlywell.com, personal communication. September 8, 2020.

North American Menopause Society. "What is Hormone Testing?" Accessed August 2020. https://www.menopause.org/publications/clinical-practice-materials/bioidentical-hormone-therapy/what-is-hormone-testing-.

Can my doctor test me for endometriosis?
American College of Obstetricians and Gynecologists. "Endometriosis" (January 2019). https://www.acog.org/patient-resources/faqs/gynecologic-problems/endometriosis.

ACOG. "Management of Endometriosis" (July 2010). https://www.acog.org/clinical/clinical-guidance/practice-bulletin/articles/2010/07/management-of-endometriosis.

I'm trans/nonbinary/gender diverse—do I still need to go to a gynecologist?
American College of Obstetricians and Gynecologists. "Health Care for Transgender Individuals" (December 2011). https://www.acog.org/clinical/clinical-guidance/committee-opinion/articles/2011/12/health-care-for-transgender-individuals.

Possibly Pregnant

If my partner pulled out, can I still get pregnant?
Bedsider. "Withdrawal." Accessed August 2020. https://www.bedsider.org/methods/withdrawal.

Piper, Yvonne. "5 Myths about Pulling Out, Busted." Bedsider (December 11, 2013). https://www.bedsider.org/features/310-5-myths-about-pulling-out-busted.

Raine-Bennett, Tina. "Pulling Out: The Kung Fu of Contraception." Bedsider (February 28, 2011). https://www.bedsider.org/features/93-pulling-out-the-kung-fu-of-contraception.

If there is semen on my partner's hand when he fingers me, can I get pregnant?
Connecticut Children's. "Can You Get Pregnant From Fingering?" Accessed August 2020. https://www.connecticutchildrens.org/health-library/en/teens/fgrng-pregnancy.

Kendall. "Can I Get Someone Pregnant if I Have Semen (Cum) on My Finger and Touch Her Vagina?" Planned Parenthood (October 23, 2013). https://www.plannedparenthood.org/learn/teens/ask-experts/can-i-get-someone-pregnant-if-i-have-semen-cum-on-my-finger-and-touch-her-vagina.

Oops! I forgot to use protection and had sex—what now?
American College of Obstetricians and Gynecologists. "Emergency Contraception" (September 2015). https://www.acog.org/clinical/clinical-guidance/practice-bulletin/articles/2015/09/emergency-contraception.

"Emergency Contraception Pills ('Morning After Pills')." The Emergency Contraception Website. Princeton University. Accessed March 17, 2020. https://ec.princeton.edu/info/ecp.html.

Planned Parenthood. "What's the ella Morning-After Pill?" Accessed March 17, 2020. https://www.plannedparenthood.org/learn/morning-after-pill-emergency-contraception/whats-ella-morning-after-pill.

World Health Organization. "Emergency contraception" (February 2, 2018). https://www.who.int/news-room/fact-sheets/detail/emergency-contraception.

How do I get the morning-after pill or other types of emergency contraception?

Davies, Connor. "The Girl's Guide to Getting Emergency Contraception." Bedsider (March 29, 2016). https://www.bedsider.org/features/363-the-girl-s-guide-to-getting-emergency-contraception.

Shye, Ronilee. "Plan B, A to Z: Everything You Need to Know About Emergency Contraception." GoodRx (January 2, 2019). https://www.goodrx.com/blog/plan-b-a-to-z-everything-you-need-to-know-about-emergency-contraception.

Does taking emergency contraception more than once mess up my body?

American College of Obstetricians and Gynecologists. "Emergency Contraception" (September 2015). https://www.acog.org/clinical/clinical-guidance/practice-bulletin/articles/2015/09/emergency-contraception.

ACOG. "Emergency Contraception" (August 2019). https://www.acog.org/patient-resources/faqs/contraception/emergency-contraception.

I'm pregnant—and I don't know who the father is. When can I find out?

American College of Obstetricians and Gynecologists. "Prenatal Diagnostic Testing for Genetic Disorders" (May 2016). https://www.acog.org/clinical/clinical-guidance/practice-bulletin/articles/2016/05/prenatal-diagnostic-testing-for-genetic-disorders.

Donnenfeld, Alan E. and Elizabeth S. Panke. "What to Do When Your Patient Wants Prenatal Paternity Testing." *Contemporary OB/GYN* (April 15, 2004). https://www.contemporaryobgyn.net/view/what-do-when-your-patient-wants-prenatal-paternity-testing.

Society for Maternal-Fetal Medicine. "Risks of Chorionic Villus Sampling and Amniocentesis." Accessed August 2020. https://www.smfm.org/publications/156-risks-of-chorionic-villus-sampling-and-amniocentesis.

Society for Maternal-Fetal Medicine Publications Committee. "Prenatal Aneuploidy Screening Using Cell-Free DNA." *American Journal of Obstetrics & Gynecology* (June 2015): 711-716. https://www.ajog.org/article/S0002-9378(15)00324-5/pdf.

How do I know if I am fertile or not?

American College of Obstetricians and Gynecologists. "Evaluating Infertility" (January 2020). https://www.acog.org/patient-resources/faqs/gynecologic-problems/evaluating-infertility.

Practice Committee of the American Society for Reproductive Medicine. "Testing and Interpreting Measures of Ovarian Reserve: A Committee Opinion." *Fertility and Sterility* 114, no. 6 (December 2020): 1151-57. https://www.asrm.org/globalassets/asrm/asrm-content/news-and-publications/practice-guidelines/for-non-members/testing_and_interpreting_measures_of_ovarian_reserve.pdf.

INDEX

ABOUT THE AUTHOR

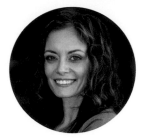

DR. JENNIFER LINCOLN is a board-certified OB-GYN who currently practices as an OB hospitalist and an International Board Certified Lactation Consultant (IBCLC) in Portland, Oregon. Dr. Lincoln loves using social media to provide evidence-based, easy-to-digest health information while busting the (many) myths surrounding vaginal and reproductive health. She believes that breaking down the shame and stigma surrounding our bodies is the best way to become informed and empowered. She is married to a pediatrician, and together they have two young boys (who will definitely be reading this book at some point).

Instagram: @drjenniferlincoln
TikTok: @drjenniferlincoln
Website: drjenniferlincoln.com

ABOUT THE ILLUSTRATOR

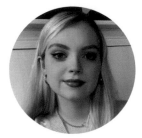

CHARLOTTE WILLCOX is an illustrator and designer from Hampshire, United Kingdom. Charlotte holds a degree in graphic arts, specializing in illustration, from the University of Southampton. She is passionate about using art as her voice to discuss important topics such as intersectional feminism, body positivity, and tackling the taboos surrounding periods.

Instagram: @charlotte.illustrates
Website: charlotteillustrates.com